Legal Issues in Sports Medicine

Healthcare providers in any setting face potential liability risks and legal challenges every day. All healthcare providers face issues such as developing strategies to mitigate those risks and creating proactive policies to reduce liability and provide better care for patients. This text presents an overview of legal issues, principles, and case law specific to athletic training and sports medicine.

Legal Issues in Sports Medicine provides an overview of legal issues and concepts for those entering or practicing in a sports medicine setting. The text addresses topics including risk management, assumption of risk, discrimination, and what to expect in the event of a lawsuit. *Legal Issues in Sports Medicine* is written for healthcare providers and students.

The authors have extensive experience in the clinical practice of athletic training, administration, and teaching on both national and international stages. This author's text comes from the perspective of years spent in the clinic and classroom and significant time in courtrooms. This book is a starting point for students of legal issues in athletic healthcare and provides a solid foundation for practice.

Greg Gardner is a clinical professor of athletic training at the University of Tulsa, USA. Dr Gardner has served as a consultant to numerous athletic training education programs in the USA as well as in Jordan and Ireland. He serves as a member of the accreditation committee for ARTI (Athletic Rehabilitators and Therapists of Ireland). He received the Sayers J. Bud Miller Outstanding Educator Award from the National Athletic Trainers' Association.

Jeff G. Konin, PhD, is a founder and partner in The Rehberg Konin Group, which specializes in sports medicine expert services and risk management. He is a clinical professor and the director of the Doctor of Athletic Training program at Florida International University in Miami, Florida, USA. Dr Konin is the co-editor of the book titled "Becoming an Expert Witness in Health Care and Litigation," and he is a member of the NATA Hall of Fame while holding Fellow status in the NATA, ACSM, and NAP organizations.

Nicole A. Wilkins, EdD, serves as the director of clinical education and director of the Henneke Center for Academic Fulfillment at The University of Tulsa, USA. With expertise in equity-minded education and leadership, faculty development, and interprofessional collaboration, she has contributed extensively to advancing athletic training practices through her research and mentorship.

Legal Issues in Sports Medicine

Greg Gardner, Jeff G. Konin, and Nicole A. Wilkins

Routledge
Taylor & Francis Group
NEW YORK AND LONDON

Designed cover image: Getty images

First published 2025
by Routledge
605 Third Avenue, New York, NY 10158

and by Routledge
4 Park Square, Milton Park, Abingdon, Oxon, OX14 4RN

Routledge is an imprint of the Taylor & Francis Group, an informa business

ISBN: 978-1-04102-595-5 (hbk)
ISBN: 978-1-63822-063-3 (pbk)
ISBN: 978-1-00352-482-3 (ebk)

DOI: 10.4324/9781003524823

Typeset in Times New Roman
by Apex CoVantage, LLC

Greg Gardner: For Jack, Emma, Jake, Madilyn, Joe, Malerie, and Lorelei. Being your Pop is the best thing ever!

Jeff Konin: To all of my legal-minded friends, Key West or bust.

Nicole Wilkins: For Bruce....Always. And to my own *West Wing:* my chosen family that embodies loyalty, wit, and the relentless drive to tackle What's Next?

Contents

About the Authors   viii
Acknowledgments   ix

1 Introduction   1

2 Framework for Legal Concepts in Athletic Training   6

3 Relating Ethical Issues to Legal Issues   17

4 Informed Consent   28

5 Standard of Care   43

6 Documentation in Athletic Training   48

7 Setting-Specific Legal Cases   54

8 Clinical Topic-Specific Cases   68

9 Discrimination   79

10 Risk Management   89

11 I Am Being Sued. Now What?   96

Index   *105*

About the Authors

Greg Gardner is a clinical professor of athletic training at the University of Tulsa, USA. Dr Gardner has served as a consultant to numerous athletic training education programs in the USA as well as internationally in Jordan and Ireland. He currently serves as a member of the accreditation committee for ARTI (Athletic Rehabilitators and Therapists of Ireland). Gardner was inducted into the Mid-America Athletic Trainers Association Hall of Fame in 2013, the Oklahoma Athletic Trainers Association Hall of Fame in 2014, and the National Athletic Trainers Association Hall of Fame in 2020. In June of 2020 he received the Sayers J. Bud Miller Outstanding Educator Award from the National Athletic Trainers' Association.

Dr Jeff G. Konin is a founder and partner in The Rehberg Konin Group, which specializes in sports medicine expert services and risk management. He is a clinical professor and the director of the Doctor of Athletic Training program at Florida International University in Miami, Florida. Dr Konin is the co-editor of the book titled "Becoming an Expert Witness in Health Care and Litigation," and he is a member of the NATA Hall of Fame while holding Fellow status in the NATA, ACSM, and NAP organizations.

Dr Nicole A. Wilkins is a leader and accomplished athletic training educator with nearly 20 years of clinical experience. She currently serves as the director of clinical education and director of the Henneke Center for Academic Fulfillment at The University of Tulsa. With expertise in equity-minded education and leadership, faculty development, and interprofessional collaboration, she has contributed extensively to advancing athletic training practices through her research and mentorship. A dedicated scholar and mentor, Dr Wilkins is committed to advancing athletic training education and shaping the future of the profession through innovative research and student-centered approaches.

Acknowledgments

As co-authors of this textbook, we extend our deepest gratitude to the many individuals who have supported us throughout this journey. We are especially thankful to the mentors, colleagues, and legal professionals whose expertise and guidance were invaluable in shaping the foundation of this work. Their dedication to advancing the profession of athletic training and fostering legal awareness has inspired and informed this text.

To the athletic trainers, educators, and students who shared their experiences and perspectives, thank you for providing the real-world context that makes this book practical and relevant. Your commitment to patient care and professional growth drives the ongoing evolution of our field.

We are also immensely grateful to our families and friends for their unwavering support, encouragement, and patience as we dedicated countless hours to this project.

Finally, we extend our appreciation to the publishers and editorial team for their partnership and expertise in transforming this vision into a comprehensive and accessible resource.

This book is a testament to the collective efforts of a community committed to advancing the legal and ethical practice of athletic training. To all who contributed, thank you for helping us make this vision a reality.

1   Introduction

Chapter Objectives: Following the completion of this chapter, the reader will:

1. Understand the purpose and scope of this text.
2. Recognize the importance of specific areas of focus presented in the text.
3. Understand how of material in the chapter, and the rest of the textbook, can be applied to different practice settings.

Introduction

In October of 2016, Logan Wood was participating in and junior high football game at North Myrtle Beach Middle School. Logan suffered a head injury but the symptoms were not recognized by the coaching staff and there was no athletic trainer present.[1] Logan was symptomatic after he was struck in the head in the first half of the game but was allowed to continue to play and even played in the second half. Sarah Wood, Logan's legal guardian, brought suit against Horry County School District alleging the school acted with gross negligence or recklessness in disregarding the school district's athletic department policy on removing students with concussion signs from participation. The Horry County Court of Common Pleas agreed that the actions of the school were negligent and awarded the family 600,000 dollars.

In the state of Washington in July of 2018, 16-year-old Allen Harris was participating in pre-season football practice when he collapsed.[2] Allen died later that day afternoon. An autopsy determined Allen had a condition known as hypertrophic cardiac myopathy. At that time, Washington state law required school districts to develop an emergency action plan, including using an AED, and train employees to initiate the plan. The Harris family filed a lawsuit against Federal Way Public Schools alleging the negligent actions of the coaches present at practice that day were the cause of Allen's death. The court agreed and the family was awarded damages.

DOI: 10.4324/9781003524823-1

A Word on WHY This Book is Important

Both Wood's and Allen's cases serve to underscore the significant level of risk associated with any physical activity as well as the importance of proper intervention and actions in the event of injury to participants. Both cases also support the importance of studying the legal aspects of providing healthcare in athletics. This text is intended to facilitate such a study as well as provide opportunities and exercises to encourage critical thinking in areas related to the legal liability encountered by any sports healthcare delivery team.

Sports medicine teams or athletic healthcare teams all share a common legal obligation to their patients/clients/athletes, regardless of where that patient or athlete is seen or treated. Whether the patient or athlete is treated in a clinic or on a soccer field, the legal obligation remains unchanged. A great starting point for the study of liability in sports medicine or athletic training is an examination of the basic elements of negligence, duty, breach, cause, and harm. This text will use case law to present and clarify relevant legal concepts. As an example, in the previous cases both school systems clearly had a duty to provide adequate emergency care of students. It is also readily apparent that there was a breach of that duty. A direct causal relationship between the actions, or rather a failure to act, of the coaching staff in both cases was clearly established in court. Both Wood and Allen, as will other cases presented in this text, can be used to present and explain legal issues that should be foundational knowledge for sports medicine team members.

Beyond the legal duty, clinicians and administrators have clearly delineated ethical responsibility to the patients or athletes. Athletic trainers, physicians, and other members of the sports medicine team practice within their respective ethical frameworks. Athletic trainers must work within the National Athletic Trainers Association Code of Ethics[3] and the Board of Certification Standards of Professional Practice.[4] Likewise, physicians work within an ethical framework as part of the team providing athletic healthcare.[5] All clinicians providing healthcare to the patient/client/athlete in sports are ethically obligated to provide care that meets current standards of practice and to do so in a safe environment, free of bias or discrimination. It is an obligation as old as the practice of medicine, originating from the Hippocratic Oath.

That legal and ethical obligations exist is well established. Professional obligations to employers, colleagues, and patients also exist.[6] Although the primary responsibility of any clinician is to their patient, clinicians have a professional responsibility to their employers in addition to legal and ethical obligations.[7] This responsibility should be extended to colleagues the clinician works with. Clinicians are obligated to practice using the most current standards of care, communicate and interact professionally, and do so to safeguard against any liability risks encountered by the clinician group. This text will help students become more aware of those legal, professional, and ethical responsibilities.

A Word on the WHAT This Book Covers

Topics presented in this text were selected to present a broad range of legal risks that may be encountered by clinicians providing athletic healthcare services. Readers should be reminded that while this text is based on long-established medicolegal tenets, new issues will arise, and clinicians will encounter new legal challenges in their practice. It is incumbent upon clinicians to remain vigilant and current as new legal issues or rulings emerge.

To assist in this introductory study of medicolegal issues, topics selected include legal terminology, medical documentation, setting-specific issues, specific clinic topics, risk management, ethical issues that become legal issues, discrimination, and what to expect when and if you do get sued.

Legal terminology can be complicated and very much like a foreign language. In fact, many legal terms are Latin terms but are still in common use today. For example, the term respondeat superior can be loosely translated to "let the master answer." Respondeat superior represents a critically important concept in the medicolegal realm. Simply put, it means you will be responsible for the actions of your employees, or those you supervise. The existence of this doctrine makes your obligation to ensure those you hire are qualified, competent, and providing high-quality healthcare services a very real burden, one that has been legally established and recognized in courts for ages.

Medical document is an area that has the potential to either rescue the clinician charged with failing to deliver an appropriate standard of care or condemn the clinician by its absence. There are many cases involving medical documents that are either below standard or, as previously stated, absent entirely. If challenged in a court case, an action that is not documented, legally, did not happen.

Ethical codes of conduct must be adhered to in professional practice. Unfortunately, unethical conduct, cared to excess, can easily escalate into legal misconduct. An immediate example is the ethical obligation to remain current in practice standards and techniques. Failing to do so is unethical. Carried a step further, failing to provide a standard of care to your patient/client/athlete immediately becomes a breach of duty and is halfway to becoming negligence.

One of the challenges in sports medicine or athletic healthcare is the variety of settings encountered by the clinician. Many of the challenges are very specific. Consider the challenges faced by a secondary school athletic trainer that is created simply by virtue of the fact that the patient/athlete is a minor. The other side of that coin could be a sports medicine team delivering healthcare to a professional athlete and encountering worker compensation or player association issues.

That clinicians must remain current in all practice areas is without question. There are, however, certain areas that are problematic for a variety of reasons. For example, much of what is known about traumatic brain injury and concussion has been learned in the past 15 years. There are many legal issues and considerations associated with head injuries, in part, because so much new knowledge is being published that guidelines and standards are somewhat fluid. The same is true for cardiac issues in athletics. Standards of practice and guidelines for general population cardiac patients are not the same for a patient that is a competitive athlete. That fact, in and of itself, presents a challenge for clinicians.

Discrimination-related issues are covered in the text as this is an area which has both ethical and legal ramifications. Clinicians practicing in educational institutions must be cognizant of issues stemming from violation of Title IX legislation. Case law involving actions that constitute sexual harassment are presented and discussed in an effort to help clinicians in developing policies and procedures that respect and protect the rights of their patients/athletes.

Risk management, as a practice, is presented in the text and should be considered a duty equal in importance to staying current in any practice area. Risk management should be considered as a proactive strategy as opposed to reactive. Damage control is a woefully inadequate step in protecting your patient, yourself, and your employer. It is infinitely better to develop plans, policies, and procedures to prevent the event from happening than it is to strategize on how to react when it does!

The best efforts of a clinician to avoid litigation may fail, and the issue may end up in court. In that event, a chapter in the text covers what happens in the event of a lawsuit. Forewarned is forearmed and it behooves clinicians to be prepared for what to expect in a courtroom. Most clinicians have no idea what to expect when they enter the courtroom. Going into a lawsuit totally uninformed, having no idea what to expect, is unwise and potentially very dangerous. Without question, it is best to conduct your practice in a manner to avoid litigation, but if the unfortunate does happen, it is highly advisable to know as much as possible about the process and what to expect when it does happen.

A Word on HOW the Text Covers the Material

Each chapter of the text is preceded by chapter objectives which chart the content course of that chapter. The three authors of the text, each writing different chapters, have developed and written the chapter from the perspective of it being used in a classroom. The chapter objectives should be used to orient you to the content and help you start the process of learning the material.

Case law cited in each of the chapters serves as both a foundation for the concepts that are presented as well as providing clear examples of those concepts in practical application. Most of the cases are well established and will likely stand the test of time because they are established and represent significant points of law. One example is the case of Kleinknecht v. Gettysburg[8], which clearly establishes the existence of a duty, owed by a university to a student athlete in that university. Kleinknecht also serves as an excellent example of how policies and procedures could be developed and implemented to help the university protect the student athlete and also manage the risks incurred in operating and college athletic program. Case law is the foundation of much of this textbook and familiarity with these cases should be fundamental for all entering athletic training or any profession within the sports medicine realm.

Each chapter contains case studies that provide an opportunity to test run newly gained knowledge. Case studies present scenarios in which critical thinking and application are required in order to resolve the situation. Some of the case studies are loosely based on the existing case law. Some of the case studies are derived from the personal experience of the author. All are designed to help you dive deeper into the content and facilitate in-depth consideration of the topic.

References

1. Grossly Negligent: Failing to Staff an Athletic Trainer and Failing to Pull Visibly Concussed Middle School Football Player Results in Verdict Against South Carolina School District. *Sports Litigation Alert*. Accessed August 29, 2024. https://sportslitigationalert.com/grossly-negligent-failing-to-staff-an-athletic-trainer-and-failing-to-pull-visibly-concussed-middle-school-football-player-results-in-verdict-against-south-carolina-school-district/
2. Harris v. Federal Way Public Schools. *Findlaw*. 2022. Accessed July 29, 2024. https://caselaw.findlaw.com/court/wa-court-of-appeals/2163968.html
3. nata-code-of-ethics.pdf. Accessed December 29, 2023. https://www.nata.org/sites/default/files/nata-code-of-ethics.pdf
4. boc-standards-of-professional-practice-2018–20180619.pdf. Accessed March 18, 2023. https://www.bocatc.org/system/document_versions/versions/154/original/boc-standards-of-professional-practice-2018–20180619.pdf?1529433022
5. Koller DL. Team Physicians, Sports Medicine, and the Law. *Clinics in Sports Medicine*. 2016;35(2):245–255. doi:10.1016/j.csm.2015.10.005
6. Beauchamp TL, Childress JF. *Principles of Biomedical Ethics*. 7th ed. Oxford University Press; 2013.
7. H−225.950 AMA Principles for Physician Employment. *AMA*. Accessed July 29, 2024.
8. *Kleinknecht v. Gettysburg College*, 786 F. Supp. 449 (M.D. Pa. 1992).

2 Framework for Legal Concepts in Athletic Training

Chapter Objectives: Following the completion of this chapter, the reader will:

1. Define and explain key legal terminology in athletic training.
2. Understand the roles of governing agencies and regulatory bodies at the state and federal levels.
3. Identify strategies to mitigate risk in clinical practice to minimize the chances of litigation.

Introduction

With the adoption of the 2020 Commission on Accreditation of Athletic Training Education[1] (CAATE) standards, the volume and magnitude of curricular content that must be taught and assessed in athletic training education programs have grown to reflect the evolution of the profession itself. While the scope of the educational content has widened to reflect the additional skills athletic trainers can perform in clinical practice, the emphasis on material related to legal liability, risk management, and healthcare administration continues to shrink. In fact, only two of the 94 required programmatic standards for professional programs identify concepts related to legal liability or legal aspects of the profession[1]. This lack of emphasis is further reflected in the Board of Certification Practice Analysis[2, 3], which shows a 5% reduction in questions on content contained within Domain V (Healthcare Administration and Professional Responsibility) Board of Certification Exam (n=10). Additionally, upon graduation and becoming a credentialed athletic trainer, opportunities to seek out additional training on legal liability and risk management are limited.

Which begs the question: If the content is not emphasized in the educational curriculum and there are limited resources for credentialed providers to enhance their knowledge, where are people getting their information from? Research suggests that the general public's impressions and perceptions of the legal system were highly influenced by television shows such as "Law and Order" and "CSI"[4-6]. Additionally, websites such as Legal Zoom[7] and Legal Shield[8] can be helpful for individuals seeking legal counsel and other legal services.

As such, the intention of this chapter is to provide clarity to the somewhat confounding key legal definitions. Additionally, this chapter provides an overview of

DOI: 10.4324/9781003524823-2

foundational information and key legal concepts while offering the reader practical strategies to reduce their risk of legal liability.

Overview of Regulatory Requirements in Athletic Training

Before diving into the specific legal terms and principles presented in the remainder of this chapter, it is important to review foundational information that serves as the framework for compliance with legal and regulatory requirements in athletic training.

Credentialing and Regulatory Processes

Ensuring that healthcare providers have obtained and maintained appropriate licensing and credentialing is essential as a risk mitigation strategy. Not only does it confirm that individuals have met the established professional standards of education and training, but it also provides safeguards for patient safety while presenting a framework for ethical and competent clinical practice. In athletic training, these professional standards are regulated and monitored both through the BOC[9] and individual state licensing boards. As with other healthcare providers, the exact scope of practice and duties of athletic trainers can vary from state to state, making it critical that both certified athletic trainers and athletic training students are familiar with their individual state practice acts. In 2018, the Sports Medicine Licensure Clarity Act[10–12] was signed into law, which provides legal protections to athletic trainers when they travel across state lines with their athletes. This act permits athletic trainers to offer the same medical services in a secondary state as they do in their home state, provided that secondary state's licensure requirements are similar to those of their home state[10–12].

At the time of publication of this text, all 50 states and the District of Columbia have some form of regulation in place related to the practice of athletic training[13]. Regulatory requirements can vary from state to state, and the most up-to-date information can be found on the BOC website[14]. All states, except for Hawaii and California, now utilize licensure as their chosen form of state regulation[14], which comes on the heels of both South Carolina and New York updating their practice acts in 2023 to move from a certification model to a licensure model[15]. Additionally, in September 2024, California made huge strides in its regulatory efforts with the passage of *AB796 Title Protection for Athletic Trainers*[13, 16], which prohibits individuals from calling themselves an athletic trainer or using similar titles unless they are certified by the BOC or have graduated from an accredited athletic training program.

Governing Agencies

The Strategic Alliance[17] is composed of four groups: the National Athletic Trainers' Association[18] (NATA), the Board of Certification, Inc.[9] (BOC), the Commission on the Accreditation of Athletic Training Education[19] (CAATE), and the NATA Research & Education Foundation[20] (NATA Foundation). While these four organizations work in collaboration with each other, the focus of each arm of the Strategic Alliance serves a specific and unique set of shareholders.

Having a clear understanding of the role of each of the arms of the Strategic Alliance ensures that issues related to the profession are addressed in a timely manner by the appropriate agency. For example, complaints related to violations of membership standards and professional ethics should be reported to the NATA, whereas complaints related to violations of practice standards should be reported to the BOC.

Key Legal Terms

In addition to understanding the regulatory framework previously outlined, athletic trainers need a strong comprehension of several legal terms and principles that impact their responsibilities and roles as healthcare providers.

Standard of Care: Defined as "the uniform standard of behavior upon which the theory of negligence is based,"[21] the standard of care in athletic training is a comprehensive set of guidelines and recommendations that specify what constitutes providing appropriate healthcare. Members of the NATA can access standard of care checklists for the secondary school[22] and collegiate[23] levels to ensure compliance with the accepted standards within athletic training, identify current baseline measurements, and assess quality assurance for services provided.

Scope of Practice: As defined by the American Medical Association[24], scope of practice refers to the activities a licensed person is legally able to perform. In healthcare, the scope of practice is outlined in individual state practice acts, and the provisions outlined can vary from state to state. Further discussion of the scope of practice can be found in Chapter 5 of this textbook.

Liability: Simply defined, liability is holding a party legally responsible for something, which can include actions, inactions, or the actions of people they are legally responsible for[25]. This includes covering athletic events[26] and patient care[27, 28]. Members of the NATA have access to the NATA Liability Toolkit[29] which can be useful to employees, supervisors, and legal counsel to identify areas of exposure to liability risk in their workplace setting.

Informed Consent: Defined as "consent given only after full disclosure of what is being consented to," informed consent in healthcare refers to patient's being made aware of the nature and risks of a medical procedure to be rendered[30]. Further discussion of the impact of informed consent can be found in Chapter 4 of this textbook.

Negligence and Malpractice

Understanding the legal terms defined earlier is important; however, it is more imperative for athletic trainers to understand the consequences of failing to adhere to the accepted professional standards and scope of practice. The following section highlights concepts related to negligence and malpractice and provides strategies to reduce the risk of negligence lawsuits.

Tort: A tort is a legal wrongdoing that rises to the level in which the courts become involved to provide a remedy, usually in the form of monetary damages[31, 32]. Torts fall into three general categories—intentional torts (i.e., battery and assault), negligent torts (i.e., act of omission), and strict liability torts (i.e., product liability, possession crimes, and statutory rape)[32]. While many of these types of torts can be present within the profession of athletic training, negligent torts are most reported[33, 34] and can encompass issues such as medical malpractice, improper medical clearance, and failure to have an emergency action plan[35, 36].

Negligence: Negligence is defined as the failure to exercise the standard of care[37] that a reasonably prudent person would exercise in like circumstances[38]. In healthcare, this is also referred to as medical malpractice and can vary in severity from technical errors that occur during medical procedures to misdiagnosis of a disease[35].

There are five fundamental components that must be established and proven in a negligence case[37, 39] and include an established duty to care, breach of that duty by the defendant, harm caused to the plaintiff, proof that the defendant's actions are the proximate cause of harm to the plaintiff and that the defendant's actions are cause-in-fact of harm to the plaintiff[37, 39].

Established Duty to Care: It is the responsibility of the athletic trainer to provide sound healthcare that protects the health and safety of their athletes and patients[27] and should be viewed as similar to that of the physician-patient relationship. Duty to care standards are outlined in the BOC Standards of Professional Practice[40] and are regularly reviewed and updated to ensure that these standards are consistent with contemporary healthcare standards and practices.

Breach of Duty: A breach of duty arises when an athletic trainer or medical provider deviates from the accepted standard of care. Breach of duty can occur in the form of *misfeasance*[41] (improper and unlawful execution of an act that in itself is lawful), an act of *omission/nonfeasance*[42] (a failure to do something or the neglect to perform what the law requires), or an act of *commission/malfeasance*[43] (the doing of an illegal and unlawful act).

The following examples are athletic training specific and can help provide a clearer understanding of the concepts in clinical practice.

Misfeasance: An athletic trainer leaves a moist heat pack on an athlete for too long, resulting in burning the athlete's skin.

Nonfeasance: An athletic trainer witnesses an athlete suffering a head injury but fails to perform an assessment or follow accepted guidelines for the management of concussions as outlined in the NATA Position Statement[44].

Malfeasance: An athletic trainer knowingly administers expired medications to their patients, resulting in adverse side effects to the medications.

Harm Caused to Plaintiff: Harm is typically thought of in terms of bodily harm or harm to physical property[37, 39]. Additionally, some states will take into account the impact of emotional distress as a form of harm to the plaintiff[37].

Proof of Proximate Cause of Harm: To satisfy this criterion in a negligence case, the plaintiff must demonstrate that the defendant's breach of duty directly caused their harm[37]. While the burden of proof falls to the plaintiff to demonstrate the existence of damages[27], if the plaintiff engages in behaviors that increase the risk of harm, the defendant's liability may be limited or negated[37].

Cause-in-Fact of Harm: This final element for a negligence case creates a cause-and-effect relationship, in that the plaintiff would have not suffered harm had it not been for the defendant's conduct[38].

It should be noted that as tort and negligence laws have evolved, there has been a shift away from the previous four-criterion approach which combined the last two elements under the category of cause. While the content addressed in the proximal cause of harm and cause-in-fact of harm are similar in nature, the adoption of a five-criterion approach that separates the two allows for key details, such as identifying a cause-and-effect relationship, to be extrapolated and considered[39]. For the defendant to be found guilty of negligence, all five criteria must be established and proven[27].

Federal Regulations

The Health Insurance Portability and Accountability Act[45] (HIPAA) and the Family Educational Rights and Privacy Act[46] (FERPA) are federal acts that regulate the confidentiality and privacy of patient's health and educational records, respectively. These acts not only set limits on who has access to these records but also empower the individual to decide how this information is disclosed and used. It is imperative that athletic trainers have policies and procedures in place to protect these documents and ensure compliance with confidentiality. Furthermore, it is critical that these policies and procedures are reflective of maintaining confidentiality with the growing use of electronic medical records and the increasing presence of social media. While content related to HIPAA and FERPA is taught and assessed in athletic training programs[1], research shows that there is still a disconnect in the application of this content in clinical practice. A 2018 study by Winkelmann et al.[47] found that athletic training students lack sound e-professionalism practices when it comes to social media and may not be fully aware of the risks of potential HIPAA violations when posting to social media. Strategies for confidentiality compliance, specifically related to documentation practices, can be found in Chapter 6 of this textbook.

Risk Management and Liability Reduction Strategies

As previously mentioned, it is important that athletic trainers engage in strategies to minimize the chance for legal action. At a minimum, athletic trainers should strictly adhere to their state practice acts and follow the updated guidelines established by the BOC for professional practice[40], maintain confidentiality with HIPAA and FERPA compliance, and ensure that informed consent is obtained prior to initiating and rendering treatment. Additional risk management strategies include, but are not limited to:

<u>Documentation:</u> Clear, concise, and accurate documentation practices are essential in healthcare. In the litigious society we live in, it is more important than

ever for athletic trainers to ensure they are engaging in sound documentation practices. Members of the NATA can access the "Best Practice Guidelines for Athletic Training Documentation"[48] which offers strategies for implementing documentation practices that are in alignment with established best practices. A more in-depth discussion on documentation can be found in Chapter 6 of this textbook.

Emergency Action Plans (EAPs): An emergency action plan is a detailed written plan that outlines the preparation, response, and on-site management of medical emergencies in the prehospital setting[49]. The NATA released an updated statement in 2024 that provides contemporary guidelines for the development and implementation of EAPs[49]. It is crucial that EAPs are venue specific, reviewed and practiced annually with all key stakeholders, and discussed before all competitions as part of the pre-game medical timeout[49]. The importance of having an EAP was recently demonstrated with the passage of Riley's Rule[50] in the state of Oklahoma. This act was signed into law in 2023 and ensures that EAPs are developed and posted for each facility where athletic practices, events, or activities are held[50].

Good Samaritan Law: Protections under this law are provided to "one who renders voluntary aid without compensation to a person who is injured or in danger"[51]. All 50 states provide protection under the Good Samaritan Law, which were designed to protect healthcare providers from liability for rendering services outside of their normal clinical environment[52]. However, providers must provide care that falls within their scope of practice and exercise a reasonable standard of care to ensure that they remain protected under this law[52].

Liability Insurance: Athletic trainers should invest in liability insurance that goes beyond employer-sponsored coverage, especially those that seek out PRN or contract work outside of their normal employment. Employer-sponsored coverage does not typically provide coverage for those types of events[53], and contract work sites like Go4[54] require proof of liability insurance to be hired. There are numerous companies that offer liability insurance coverage for athletic trainers, and members of the NATA can receive a discounted policy through partner companies[53].

Application in Clinical Practice

Over the last decade, negligence cases involving athletic trainers have become more high-profile and public-facing, drawing attention from the media and the public. Additionally, some of these high-profile cases may result in a settlement agreement between parties to avoid a trial. The cases listed subsequently represent a handful of negligence cases involving athletic trainers and serve as a reminder for athletic trainers to adhere to established legal and ethical standards in clinical practice to ensure the health and safety of their patients.

Feleccia v. Lackawanna College[55,56] *(2019)*: Lackawanna College hired two recent graduates as athletic trainers in 2009, knowing they had not passed the BOC examination or obtained Pennsylvania licensure. Upon discovering they were not properly credentialed, the college changed their titles to "first responders" but kept their responsibilities the same. After two student athletes were seriously injured during practice, the athletes sued, alleging the college was grossly negligent in failing to hire qualified medical personnel.

Pinson v. State[27, 57] *(1996)*: This case highlights the athletic trainer's failure to properly report key symptoms of a head injury. After Michael Pinson reported a head blow and collapsed unconscious for ten minutes, the trainer failed to communicate symptom severity to the hospital physician and ignored medical advice for Pinson to abstain from football for a week. Despite Pinson's ongoing headaches, the trainer reported him as symptom-free, leading to his premature return to play. A month later, Pinson collapsed again and required surgery for chronic subdural hematomas, resulting in permanent neurological damage. The trainer unsuccessfully argued that negligence elements, including duty to disclose and breach of duty, were not responsible for Pinson's injuries.

Williams v. Athletico[58] *(2017)*: This case also demonstrates the failure of the athletic trainer to properly assess and address concussion symptoms in an athlete. Drew Williams suffered what was reported as a "significant blow to the head" during a football game and was not evaluated for a possible concussion at the time of injury. He was allowed to continue playing in the game, sustaining several additional hits to the head, and would eventually be removed from the game in the fourth quarter. The court found that the athletic trainer's actions were negligent based on the lack of adherence to established standards of care[58].

Conclusion

It is imperative that athletic trainers understand and apply the key legal definitions and principles discussed in this chapter. While these topics represent only a small portion of BOC examination questions, the cases highlighted, and others like it, demonstrate the real-world implications of not following established standards of care and maintaining documented professional standards. By adopting proactive risk management strategies, such as ensuring proper documentation and following accepted standards of care, athletic trainers can significantly reduce the risk of legal action.

References

1. Commission on Accreditation of Athletic Training Education. *Standards and Procedures for Accreditation of Professional Programs in Athletic Training.* 2024. Accessed October 6, 2024. https://caate.net/Portals/0/Standards_and_Procedures_Professional_Programs.pdf?ver=01iHqzdBAW0IsGARUc-19Q%3d%3d
2. BOCadmin. *BOC Practice Analysis, 8th Edition May Impact Your Education Program.* Board of Certification for the Athletic Trainer. February 15, 2023. Accessed October 12, 2024. https://bocatc.org/newsroom/boc-practice-analysis-8th-edition-may-impact-your-education-program/
3. Board of Certification for the Athletic Trainer. *Content Outline for Practice Analysis.* 8th ed. Published online March 2023. https://bocatc.org/wp-content/uploads/2024/01/boc-pa8-content-outline-20230109-1.pdf

4. Journal ABA. Law & Order's Prime-time Formula Shaped a Generation's Understanding of the Legal System. *ABA Journal.* Accessed October 12, 2024. https://www.abajournal.com/magazine/article/LawAndOrders-prime-time-formula-shaped-a-generations-understanding-of-the-legal-system
5. Parker S. The Portrayal of the American Legal System in Prime Time Television Crime Dramas. *Elon Journal of Undergraduate Research in Communications.* 2013;4(1). Accessed October 12, 2024. http://www.inquiriesjournal.com/articles/794/the-portrayal-of-the-american-legal-system-in-prime-time-television-crime-dramas
6. Sutton DL, Britts M, Landman M. Law and Order and the American Criminal Justice System. *Kinema: A Journal for Film and Audiovisual Media.* Published online November 20, 2000. doi:10.15353/kinema.vi.907
7. LegalZoom: Start Your Business, Form Your LLC or INC. *LegalZoom.* Accessed October 12, 2024. https://www.legalzoom.com/
8. Online Legal Services and Legal Advice. *LegalShield.* Accessed October 12, 2024. https://www.legalshield.com/
9. Board of Certification for the Athletic Trainer. *Board of Certification for the Athletic Trainer.* Accessed October 12, 2024. https://bocatc.org/
10. Sen. Thune J [R S. S.808 - 115th Congress (2017–2018): Sports Medicine Licensure Clarity Act of 2017. July 9, 2018. Accessed October 13, 2024. https://www.congress.gov/bill/115th-congress/senate-bill/808
11. Sports Medicine Licensure Clarity Act Signed into Law. *NATA.* October 5, 2018. Accessed October 12, 2024. https://www.nata.org/nata-now/articles/2018/10/sports-medicine-licensure-clarity-act-signed-law
12. Rep. Guthrie B [R K 2. H.R.302 - 115th Congress (2017–2018): An Act to Provide Protections for Certain Sports Medicine Professionals, to Reauthorize Federal Aviation Programs, to Improve Aircraft Safety Certification Processes, and for Other Purposes. October 5, 2018. Accessed October 13, 2024. https://www.congress.gov/bill/115th-congress/house-bill/302
13. CTAdmin. Passage of Athletic Training Practice Act—Win for California. *Board of Certification for the Athletic Trainer.* October 11, 2024. Accessed October 13, 2024. https://bocatc.org/newsroom/passage-of-athletic-training-practice-act-win-for-california/
14. BOC Athletic Trainer State Regulation Map. *Board of Certification for the Athletic Trainer.* Accessed October 13, 2024. https://bocatc.org/state-regulation-map/
15. BOCadmin. South Carolina and New York Update AT Licensure Laws. *Board of Certification for the Athletic Trainer.* October 18, 2023. Accessed October 13, 2024. https://bocatc.org/newsroom/south-carolina-and-new-york-update-at-licensure-laws/
16. AB 796-CHAPTERED. Accessed October 13, 2024. https://leginfo.legislature.ca.gov/faces/billNavClient.xhtml?bill_id=202320240AB796
17. Home. *AT Strategic Alliance.* Accessed October 12, 2024. https://www.atstrategicalliance.org/
18. NATA. *NATA.* Accessed October 12, 2024. https://www.nata.org/
19. CAATE | Recognized by CHEA. Accessed October 12, 2024. https://caate.net/
20. NATA Research & Education Foundation. *Supporting and Advancing the Athletic Training Profession through Research and Education.* Accessed October 12, 2024. https://www.natafoundation.org/
21. Gifis SH. Standard of Care. In: *Barron's Dictionary of Legal Terms.* 5th ed. Barrons Educational Services; 2016.
22. National Athletic Trainers' Association. *Appropriate Medical Care Standards for Organizations Sponsoring Athletic Activity for the Secondary School Age Athlete.* Published online March 2019. https://www.nata.org/sites/default/files/nata_appropriate_medical_care_standards.pdf
23. Collegiate Standard of Care Toolkit. *NATA.* February 17, 2023. Accessed October 13, 2024. https://www.nata.org/collegiate-standard-care-collaterals

24. What Is Scope of Practice? *American Medical Association.* May 25, 2022. Accessed October 13, 2024. https://www.ama-assn.org/practice-management/scope-practice/what-scope-practice
25. liability. *LII/Legal Information Institute.* Accessed October 14, 2024. https://www.law.cornell.edu/wex/liability
26. Quandt EF, Mitten MJ, Black JS. Legal Liability in Covering Athletic Events. *Sports Health.* 2009;1(1):84–90. doi:10.1177/1941738108327530
27. Osborne B. Principles of Liability for Athletic Trainers: Managing Sport-Related Concussion. *Journal of Athletic Training.* 2001;36(3):316–321.
28. Risk and Liability. *NATA.* August 29, 2017. Accessed October 14, 2024. https://www.nata.org/practice-patient-care/risk-liability
29. NATA Liability Toolkit. *NATA Forms.* Accessed October 14, 2024. https://forms.nata.org/liability_tk?destination=my_liability_tk
30. Gifis SH. Informed Consent. In: *Barron's Dictionary of Legal Terms.* 5th ed. Barrons Educational Services; 2016.
31. Tort. In: *Merriam-Webster.* https://dictionary.law.com/Default.aspx?selected=2137
32. tort. *LII/Legal Information Institute.* Accessed October 13, 2024. https://www.law.cornell.edu/wex/tort
33. Henderson J. Why Negligence Dominates Tort. *UCLA Law Review University of California, Los Angeles School of Law.* 2002;50:377–405.
34. Abraham K. The Trouble with Negligence. *SSRN Electronic Journal.* 2000;54. doi:10.2139/ssrn.252064
35. Dahlawi S, Menezes R, Khan M, Waris A, Saifullah, Naseer M. Medical Negligence in Healthcare Organizations and Its Impact on Patient Safety and Public Health: A Bibliometric Study. *F1000Research.* 2021;10(174). doi:10.12688/f1000research.37448.1
36. Petraglia A, Bailes J, Day A. *Handbook of Neurological Sports Medicine.* Human Kinetics; 2014.
37. negligence. *LII/Legal Information Institute.* Accessed October 13, 2024. https://www.law.cornell.edu/wex/negligence
38. Merriam-Webster. *Negligence.* Merriam-Webster; 2019.
39. David G. Owen. The Five Elements of Negligence. *Hofstra Law Review.* 35(1):1671–1686.
40. Board of Certification for the Athletic Trainer. *BOC Standards of Professional Practice.* Published online 2023. Accessed October 6, 2024. https://bocatc.org/wp-content/uploads/2024/01/SOPP-2024.pdf
41. Gifis SH. Misfeasance. In: *Barron's Dictionary of Legal Terms.* 5th ed. Barrons Educational Services; 2016.
42. Gifis SH. Omission. In: *Barron's Dictionary of Legal Terms.* 5th ed. Barrons Educational Services; 2016.
43. Gifis SH. Malfeasance. In: *Barron's Dictionary of Legal Terms.* 5th ed. Barrons Educational Services; 2016.
44. Broglio SP, Register-Mihalik JK, Guskiewicz KM, Leddy JJ, Merriman A, Valovich McLeod TC. National Athletic Trainers' Association Bridge Statement: Management of Sport-Related Concussion. *Journal of Athletic Training.* 2024;59(3):225–242. doi:10.4085/1062-6050-0046.22
45. Health Insurance Portability and Accountability Act of 1996. *ASPE.* August 20, 1996. Accessed October 14, 2024. https://aspe.hhs.gov/reports/health-insurance-portability-accountability-act-1996
46. 34 CFR Part 99—Family Educational Rights and Privacy. Accessed October 14, 2024. https://www.ecfr.gov/current/title-34/subtitle-A/part-99?toc=1
47. Winkelmann ZK, Neil ER, Eberman LE. Athletic Training Students' Knowledge of Ethical and Legal Practice with Technology and Social Media. *Athletic Training Education Journal.* 2018;13(1):3–11. doi:10.4085/13013

48. Best Practice Guidelines for Athletic Training Documentation. Published online August2017.https://www.nata.org/sites/default/files/best-practice-guidelines-for-athletic-training-documentation.pdf

49. Scarneo-Miller SE, Hosokawa Y, Drezner JA, et al. National Athletic Trainers' Association Position Statement: Emergency Action Plan Development and Implementation in Sport. *Journal of Athletic Training*. 2024;59(6):570–583. doi:10.4085/1062-6050-0521.23

50. 2023 Oklahoma Statutes :: Title 70. Schools :: §70-27-104. Short title—Riley's Rule—Emergency Action Plan for Facility and Athletic Events. *Justia Law*. October15,2024.AccessedOctober14,2024.https://law.justia.com/codes/oklahoma/title-70/section-70-27-104/

51. Steven H. Gifis. Good Samaritan Law. In: *Barron's Dictionary of Legal Terms*. 5th ed. Barrons Educational Services; 2016.

52. West B, Varacallo M. Good Samaritan Laws. In: *StatPearls*. StatPearls Publishing; 2024. Accessed October 14, 2024. http://www.ncbi.nlm.nih.gov/books/NBK542176/

53. Athletic Trainers. Accessed October 14, 2024. https://www.proliability.com/content/amba/proliability/professional-liability-insurance/athletic-trainers.html

54. Home. *Go4*. Accessed October 14, 2024. https://www.go4.io/

55. *Feleccia v. Lackawanna College, et al. (Majority)*. (Supreme Court of Pennsylvania 2019). Accessed October 14, 2024. https://casetext.com/case/feleccia-v-lackawanna-coll-6/

56. Potential Expansion of Athletic Programs' Duty of Care to Student-Athletes and New Limitations to Waivers of Liability: Lessons Learned from Feleccia v. Lackawanna College. *Sports Litigation Alert*. Accessed October 14, 2024. https://sportslitigationalert.com/potential-expansion-of-athletic-programs-duty-of-care-to-student-athletes-and-new-limitations-to-waivers-of-liability-lessons-learned-from-feleccia-v-lackawanna-college/

57. *Pinson v. State*. (Court of Appeals of Tennessee 1996). https://casetext.com/case/pinson-v-state-21

58. *Williams v. Athletico, Ltd*. (Circuit Court of Cook County 2017). https://law.justia.com/cases/illinois/court-of-appeals-first-appellate-district/2017/1-16-1902.html

CLINICAL CASE STUDY

You are the head athletic trainer at a small Division 1 university. One afternoon, you are in the athletic training facility finishing up treatments when you get a frantic call from your baseball coach. He states that one of her players took a ball to the face during batting practice and needs medical attention down at the field. The baseball field is on the opposite side of campus and takes you several minutes to arrive on the scene.

When you arrive to the field, you notice the athlete sitting in the dugout holding his face. He states that during batting practice, a ball went through a hole in the screen he was standing behind. The athlete confides in you and states that the whole team knows they shouldn't use this piece of equipment as there's a hole in the screen from repeated use. The team has made repeated complaints to the coach; however, due to lack of equipment, they are forced to use the screen at practice.

The athlete's initial complaint is pain in his right eye, and you notice swelling, bruising, and what appears to be a hyphema. You decide that it is in the athlete's best interest to take him to the emergency room and decide it is quicker to take the athlete in your own personal vehicle as the hospital is less than five minutes from campus. Upon arrival to the hospital, your athlete is immediately taken back for diagnostic testing. You offer to call the athlete's parents, and he tells you that he will call them once there's more information and a treatment plan.

A week later, you get an angry phone call from your athlete's mother asking why she was not notified of her son's injury as she just received the hospital bill and had no knowledge that her son had been hurt. After a lengthy conversation, she's informed you that she's sought counsel to sue you, the baseball coach, the athletic department, and the university for negligence.

Critical Thinking Questions:

1. Given the five elements needed to prove negligence, does the mother have grounds for a case? Why or why not?
2. What specific liability risks might the athletic trainer face in this situation? How could these risks have been mitigated?
3. How might responsibility be distributed among the athletic trainer, coach, athletic department, and university? Could one party be held more accountable than others and why?

3 Relating Ethical Issues to Legal Issues

Chapter Objectives: Following the completion of this chapter, the reader will:

1. Compare the original Hippocratic Oath to modern codes of ethical behavior
2. Recognize the unique nature of the patient population and the nature of practice in sports medicine
3. Understand the basic tenets of ethics in healthcare
4. Analyze hypothetical cases and identify specific ethical tenets
5. Distinguish between codes of professional behavior established by the National Athletic Trainers Association and Board of Certification, Inc.

When Ethical Issues Become Legal Issues

The origin of ethical thought relative to medicine and healthcare is the Hippocratic Oath.[1] Although some of the language is antiquated and dated, the basic premise of the document remains sound. Specific issues within the document include confidentiality, role fidelity, beneficence, nonmaleficence, and non-discrimination.

"I swear by Apollo the physician, and Asclepius the surgeon, likewise Hygeia and Panacea, and call all the gods and goddesses to witness, that I will observe and keep this underwritten oath, to the utmost of my power and judgment.

I will reverence my master who taught me the art. Equally with my parents, will I allow him things necessary for his support, and will consider his sons as brothers. I will teach them my art without reward or agreement; and I will impart all my acquirement, instructions, and whatever I know, to my master's children, as to my own; and likewise to all my pupils, who shall bind and tie themselves by a professional oath, but to none else.

With regard to healing the sick, I will devise and order for them the best diet, according to my judgment and means; and I will take care that they

DOI: 10.4324/9781003524823-3

suffer no hurt or damage. Nor shall any man's entreaty prevail upon me to administer poison to anyone; neither will I counsel any man to do so. Moreover, I will give no sort of medicine to any pregnant woman, with a view to destroy the child. Further, I will comport myself and use my knowledge in a godly manner.

I will not cut for the stone, but will commit that affair entirely to the surgeons.

Whatsoever house I may enter, my visit shall be for the convenience and advantage of the patient; and I will willingly refrain from doing any injury or wrong from falsehood, and (in an especial manner) from acts of an amorous nature, whatever may be the rank of those who it may be my duty to cure, whether mistress or servant, bond or free.

Whatever, in the course of my practice, I may see or hear (even when not invited), whatever I may happen to obtain knowledge of, if it be not proper to repeat it, I will keep sacred and secret within my own breast. If I faithfully observe this oath, may I thrive and prosper in my fortune and profession, and live in the estimation of posterity; or on breach thereof, may the reverse be my fate!" [2]

Unfortunately, many equate ethical conduct with moral values or perhaps believe that ethics is synonymous with good or proper behavior[3] when in reality, it is often more complex than a simple moral judgment. There are codes of ethical conduct for most, if not all, healthcare professions. A perusal of these profession-specific documents or codes leads the reader back to the Hippocratic Oath.[2,3] Of specific interest within this text is how codes of ethics or ethical behavior guidelines relate to legal issues. While it is very unlikely that an action or act could be illegal but not unethical, it is very possible for an action to be unethical and still be legal. This chapter examines the interface between ethical conduct how unethical conduct can be taken to the point of becoming an illegal action.

The Unique Nature of "Sports Medicine" Practice

Consider an example where a professional football player is knocked to the ground in a manner that results in his head being forcefully slammed into the turf. When he stands up after the play he demonstrated signs of ataxia or motor incoordination.[4] His subsequent return to play served as a catalyst for the players association and the league to seek changes in the same-day return-to-play protocol. The revised protocol dictates that no player who demonstrates specific signs of a head injury may return to competition that same day.[5] This example is not used here to point the finger of blame at any individual, organization, or group. It is, however, highly illustrative of some of the unique aspects of the practice setting many athletic trainers work in. Athletic trainers very often work with patients that, given a choice, would continue to participate and compete even when injured. This is simply the nature of much of the patient population athletic trainers deal with. Even if it's merely a weekend warrior seen in a clinic, that individual is extremely motivated to continue their workout routine, compete in their next tennis tournament, or run their next half marathon. That the actions and decisions of an athletic trainer may have both immediate and far-reaching consequences for their patient must be recognized. While this fact may not directly change the expected standard of care, the nature of the practice environment and patient population create added challenges in the decision-making processes.

Regardless of the healthcare profession, there are several basic ethic tenets of healthcare ethics. Beauchamp and Childress, in what many consider the seminal text on biomedical ethics,[6] cite four major tenets of ethics within healthcare, regardless of the area of practice. These four focal points of medical ethics include autonomy, non-maleficence, beneficence, and justice. Other areas of specific interest include confidentiality, veracity, and role fidelity. However, it can be argued that all tenets of healthcare ethics are ultimately derived from autonomy, non-maleficence/beneficence, or justice.[7] In certain situations, unethical actions taken by a clinician may reach the point of being illegal or becoming a source of litigation. These are examined more closely in the following sections of this chapter.

Autonomy

Regardless of the specific field of practice, healthcare providers are taught to respect the autonomy of their patients. Healthcare practitioners must respect the fact that their patients must become a part of medical or treatment decisions that are made. Beauchamp and Childress formally define autonomy as "personal rule of self while being free both controlling interferences from others and personal limitations, such as inadequate understanding."[7] That patients must be involved in the decision-making process relative to their health and well-being is irrefutable. It is notable that "inadequate understanding" is treated as a factor that can infringe upon the autonomy of a patient. If a patient does not have a clear understanding of all of the ramifications of a surgery or course of treatment, the patient is essentially being deprived of their autonomy. Taken a step further, if an athletic trainer, or any clinician for that matter, fails to completely inform a patient about those ramifications or risks, the athletic trainer/clinician is infringing on patient autonomy.

Consider the scenario described in the opening paragraph where a professional athlete was allowed to return to play under questionable circumstances. If the player alone were allowed to make the return-to-play decision, the chances are very good that they would jump back into the game. After all, this is a professional athlete and a consenting adult. Shouldn't they be allowed to make their own decisions regarding their health? An athletic trainer overruling the player and prohibiting their return to play is what Sims[8] identifies as paternalism. Paternalism is when the athletic trainer or therapist believes, based upon their professional judgment, the decision being made by the patient is not, medically, in their best interests. Refusing to allow the athlete with the concussion to play may be paternalistic thinking, and it also may infringe on patient autonomy. Even if a paternalistic decision may violate patient autonomy, such a decision may still be the right one to make. Without question, the clinician must respect the freedom and autonomy of the patient. Autonomy and the liberty of choice must include a safe level of logical thought or reasoning on the part of the patient. In the case of the head injury, it could be argued that the player has diminished cognitive function. If that is true, holding the athlete out is not paternalistic, rather it is providing an appropriate standard of care.

A classic case from the National Football League provides a classic example of patient autonomy gone awry and demonstrates when a sufficient level of thought, knowledge, or reasoning contributed to the damage suffered by the athlete.[7] Charlie Krueger was, by all accounts, a tough player that would play through both pain and injury when he played defensive lineman for the San Francisco 49ers from 1958 to 1973, missing only a few games due to injury. Krueger suffered a torn medial collateral ligament and, at the same time, damaged his medial meniscus. While undergoing surgery to repair the damaged medial collateral ligament it was discovered that Krueger's anterior cruciate ligament was not present. It was impossible to determine when the anterior cruciate ligament was damaged initially but it was obvious during the 1963 surgery that the ligament was no longer there. According to court documents, Krueger was not informed about the damaged anterior cruciate ligament. During the 1963 season Kruger reportedly received over 50 injections to his knee. These injections consisted of a mixture of an anesthetic and a corticosteroid. After the 1963 season, Krueger was given an estimated 14 to 20 such injections each season. Charlie Krueger retired from playing for the San Francisco 49ers in 1973. In 1978 Krueger was treated for his knee pain and X-rays were taken, at which time Krueger was informed of the severity of damage to his knee.

The premise of Krueger's complaint was that he was never fully informed of how serious his knee injury was nor was he informed that he would suffer long-term damage if he continued to play football. As previously stated, Krueger was the type of player that played through both pain and injury. One could argue that even if Krueger had been fully informed about the extent of his injuries and the negative long-term effects of those injuries, he would have continued to play anyway. The fact that the information was not shared with him was never disputed. In essence, he never had the chance to make that decision because he was never fully informed.

CASE STUDY: AUTONOMY

A junior college wrestler is competing for a spot in the regional tournament when his opponent slams him into the mat headfirst. As you evaluate the injury, it is immediately obvious that he has suffered a concussion and should be taken out of the match. If he forfeits the match due to injury, it is unlikely that he will qualify for the regional tournament. Both you and the athlete are fully aware that he is being recruited by a major university with a perennial top 10 wrestling program. The athlete believes he will lose his chance for a scholarship at that school if he fails to make the regional tournament. He begs you to let him finish the match so he can earn his chance to compete in a premier program. He feels his future is on the line.

Questions to consider:

What laws or standards of ethical practice are at issue in the situation?
Does respect for patient autonomy play a role in your decision?

Beneficence/Non-Maleficence

Beneficence and non-maleficence are very closely related to ethical tenets. Beneficence simply means to do only what is good for the patient. In that sense, it's a positive or active trait. Non-maleficence means doing nothing to harm the patient. Non-maleficence is used in a negative sense, representing something you should not do. Both terms have a great deal in common but they do differ from an action perspective. Beneficence represents taking only those actions that are good for the patient while non-maleficence means not doing anything to harm the patient.

A case in which the actions of team personnel disregarded the non-maleficence principle is illustrated in a class action suit brought by the former players[9] alleged that the National Football League failed to implement a policy regulating the use of pain masking medications used to enable players to compete when injured. The alleged actions, involving several former professional football players, provide a good example of therapeutic measures taken that provided some immediate relief from pain but had potentially deleterious long-term effects. The pain medication enabled the players to continue to compete when doing so was perhaps causing permanent damage. Within this particular fact pattern, the decision to administer the pain medication was in direct conflict with the principle of non-maleficence.

At times, decisions made by athletic trainers or team physicians seem to come into direct conflict with, at least from the perspective of the athlete, what is in the best interest of the athlete. This can be the case when an athlete is disqualified from participation for a medical reason. Nicholas Knapp was a gifted high school basketball player who received a scholarship to play for Northwestern University.[10] Prior to his arrival on campus, Knapp experienced cardiac issues that were significant enough to justify implanting an internal cardioverter defibrillator (ICD). The medical staff at Northwestern carefully considered the issue, and, after a close examination of existing standards for cardiac care, disqualified Knapp from participation. In an example of applying best practices and high standards, Northwestern used the very latest position statements and documents from experts in cardiac care. Additionally, the university honored Knapp's scholarship, thereby enabling him to complete his education. Knapp sued the university for discrimination, a case which he eventually lost. Rather than seeing Knapp in a negative light, he should be viewed as an athlete who simply wants to compete. As previously stated, the practice of sports medicine is different from other areas of medical practice, largely because our patient population is so highly motivated as to be, at times, challenging. In this situation, and others like it, honoring the principle of beneficence meant disqualifying an athlete from participation. Obviously, this was contradictory to what the athlete wanted to see happen. By disqualifying Knapp, the medical staff believed they were also protecting him from a potentially catastrophic cardiac event.

CASE STUDY: BENEFICENCE/NON-MALEFICENCE

The small college basketball team you work with is playing in the conference tournament. The starting point guard has been working diligently with you as you have been treating a severe case of tendonitis of her semitendinosus muscle. You become convinced that the injury has reached a point where the athlete needs to rest the injury and failing to do so may result in permanently damaging the muscle. The athlete desperately wants to continue to compete. The coach and the rest of the team, while not directly saying anything, want you to let the athlete compete, giving the team a better chance at advancing to the next round of tournament play.

Questions:

How should you use the ethical tenets of beneficence/non-maleficence to guide your decision making in this scenario?
Who is liable if the player suffers permanent injury as a result of continuing to compete?

Confidentiality

"Whatever I see or hear in the lives of my patients, whether in connection with my professional practice or not, which ought not to be spoken of outside, I will keep secret, as considering all such things to be private"[1]

Confidentiality is a common thread through most, if not all, [11] ethical codes of conduct in healthcare. The National Athletic Trainers' Association Code of Ethics specifically addresses confidentiality in its Principle 1.3 where it states

> Members shall preserve the confidentiality of privileged information and shall not release or otherwise publish in any form, including social media, such information to a third party not involved in the patient's care without a release unless required by law.[12]

It is of interest to note the verbiage stating, "unless required by law." While there are many states that have specific requirements and stipulations[13]for when you are required to breach confidentiality it is generally accepted that divulging healthcare information is appropriate if the patient is a danger to themselves or others. A good example of this would be when a healthcare provider has reason to believe a patient was physically abused by a parent, caretaker, or other person. In such a case, failing to contact appropriate authorities or make proper referrals not only is unethical but may very well be against state or federal laws, depending upon the age of the patient. It must be assumed that athletic trainers fall within the guidelines[14] of those required, by law, to report if evidence comes to light that a child (or minor) is being abused. As previously mentioned, you should follow the general rule of breaching confidentiality only when the safety or well-being of the patient or others is at risk.

CASE STUDY: CONFIDENTIALITY

As a secondary school athletic trainer you spend a lot of time with your student athletes. At times you are convinced you spend more time with them and they spend with their family! One student in particular has told you numerous times that he feels like his parents don't understand him. He confides in you that his trouble getting along with his folks is escalating, along with the pressure to succeed on the field and excel in the classroom. Everyone is pushing him so hard that he tells you he is ready to explode. He has even thought it would be better if he just "wasn't there" and has even considered taking his life. He begs you not to say anything to his parents as he's sure they will just "freak out" or "blow it all up."

Questions:

1. Is it appropriate to honor the athletes' plea for confidentiality?
2. What should you tell this athlete?
3. What specific guidelines should you follow in this particular case?

Discrimination

All codes of ethical conduct for healthcare providers include verbiage prohibiting discrimination and the Code of Ethics of the National Athletic Trainer's Association is no exception. In fact, the prohibition against discrimination appears as the first bullet point under the first principle. "Members shall render quality patient care regardless of the patient's race, religion, age, sex, ethnic or national origin, disability, health status, socioeconomic status, sexual orientation, or gender identity"[12] The NATA Code of Ethics is very intentional in identifying multiple groups of individuals should not be discriminated against. It must be acknowledged that the list is not all-inclusive. The spirit of the principle prohibits discrimination against any group or classification of patients.

Discrimination allegations on the basis of sex in athletics will often involve more than one individual and broaden to include an entire team or even an entire athletic department. Female rowing athletes at a university filed a lawsuit alleging they were discriminated against in not being provided adequate coaching and other resources, including adequate treatment for athletic injuries.[15] Title IX of the Civil Rights Act of 1964[16] makes discrimination on the basis of sex a violation of the United States Constitution. Although the original legislation went into effect in 1972, there are still many inequities involving female athletes. Forty-nine years after Title IX was enacted, female participants in the NCAA basketball tournament were expected to practice and prepare for the games with facilities and equipment that were far from adequate and, when compared to facilities and equipment provided for the men's players, were shamefully inadequate.[17] Discrimination may be overt and readily apparent but it may also be more subtle and less easily recognized. Failure to provide the same level of medical care when teams are traveling is a prime example. Athletic training staff in colleges and secondary schools are very often understaffed and forced to make choices on which teams will have an athletic trainer with them when they travel to out-of-town games. This situation is clearly not an intentional effort to discriminate against one team or another, but the impact may indeed be discriminatory.

CASE STUDY: DISCRIMINATION

Fall sports season is a busy time for you in your role as an athletic trainer at a large high school. There are a number of teams in their competitive season including volleyball, football, cross-country track, and both men's and women's soccer. When the football team has an out-of-town game that conflicts with a women's soccer team home game you are put in a difficult position. The football coach is adamant that you travel with the football game. The women's soccer team coach wants you to stay home and be available for their game.

Questions:

1. What guidelines or rules exist to help in making the decision on which game to focus on?
2. What policies could be in place to help make this situation easier to work through?

Scope of Practice/Role Fidelity

Within the Hippocratic Oath the concept of role fidelity is addressed. Role fidelity is simply knowing and respecting your scope of practice. The scope of practice for any clinician is, if the profession practiced by the clinician has a state licensure law, largely dictated by that state law. Other considerations also include what you have been taught or trained to do. A few short excerpts from a state practice law (Oklahoma) appear subsequently as an example.

435:25-5-1. Supervision

The work of the Athletic Trainer shall be done under the supervision of the team physician or consulting physician, although the physician need not be physically present at each activity of the athletic trainer nor be specifically consulted before each delegated task performed.

(c) Sound judgment.

Licensees shall accept responsibility for the exercise of sound judgment.

(1) Licensees shall not misrepresent in any manner, directly or indirectly, their skills, training, professional credentials, identity, or services.
(2) Licensees shall provide only those services for which they are qualified via education and/or experience and by pertinent legal regulatory process.
(3) Licensees shall provide services, make referrals, and seek compensation only for those services that are necessary.

The licensure law in this example further clarifies the scope of practice for athletic trainers in sub-point (2) mentioned earlier. Athletic trainers are allowed to perform only those skills they are trained in and agreed upon by their supervising physician.[18]

An experienced athletic trainer, working in a secondary school, treated a school administrator using dry needling. When another local clinician, practicing in a different profession from athletic training became aware of this, they reported the athletic trainer to the state board of medical licensure and supervision. When the situation was carefully examined by the licensure board it was determined that the athletic trainer was practicing outside of their scope of practice. The athletic trainer was, indeed, trained to use dry needling in their practice. The issue arose from the patient the athletic trainer was treating. In that particular state, athletic trainers are restricted to treating "athletes." In this particular incident, the patient was, as previously mentioned, a school administrator.[19]

A scary sidebar to the discussion of the scope of practice is that acting outside of this scope of practice will, in many cases, void any liability insurance policy the clinician may have. So in effect, jumping outside of the scope of practice not only is a violation of state law but also has the potential to leave the clinician uninsured in the event any claim of negligence results from it.

Conflict of Interest

Early in this chapter, the unique nature of the patient population treated by athletic trainers was alluded to. Patients are much more concerned about returning to competition or participation than they are about the long-term resolution of their current medical problem. This problem is compounded when a coach, organization, team, or other entity acts to pressure clinical decisions or hurry return-to-play timelines. If an athletic trainer is employed by a secondary school, university, or professional team the likelihood of this happening is significantly increased.[20] Anytime athletic trainers report to athletic administrators the potential for a conflict of interest exists. The same may be said for having the athletic trainer report to a club owner or general manager. Given the staggering amount of money involved in intercollegiate athletics[21], that athletic trainers working within this configuration are realizing more pressure is quite understandable.

The increasingly lucrative financial environment, at least for universities and broadcasting companies, has placed athletic trainers in situations where conflict of interest is an all too real possibility. Rapp and Ingersoll[22] address the potential for risk generated simply by the nature of the administrative structure of the healthcare delivery system an athletic trainer works in. When a healthcare provider reports directly to an athletic director or coach a very real risk is created. Healthcare providers should report to other healthcare providers or healthcare administrators. Any deviation from this structure immediately jeopardizes the quality of care provider in addition to placing the athletic trainer in a very difficult position of being asked to balance the health of the athlete with the performance outcome of a team. This is contrary to any code of ethics or standards or professional conduct. Reporting lines of this nature, albeit unintentional, actually create liability issues for the clinician and the employer.

References

1. Goran S. The Ethical Legacy of Hippocrates. *Scripta Medica (Brno)*. 2020;51(4):275–283.
2. Katsambas A, Marketos S. Hippocratic Messages for Modern Medicine (the Vindication of Hippocrates). *Journal of the European Academy of Dermatology and Venereology.* 2007;21(6):859–861. doi:10.1111/j.1468–3083.2007.02231.x
3. ATC GHE, ATC/L GGE, ATC APWP. *Administrative Topics in Athletic Training: Concepts to Practice.* 2nd ed. Slack Incorporated; 2016.
4. Tua Tagovailoa's Head Hits Hint at the Dangers of Repeat Brain Trauma. *Science News.* October 7, 2022. Accessed December 6, 2023. https://www.sciencenews.org/article/ tua-tagovailoa-concussion-traumatic-brain-injury-head-hit-risk
5. NFL Concussion Diagnosis and Management Protocol (PDF). *NFL.com.* Accessed December 6, 2023. https://www.nfl.com/playerhealthandsafety/resources/fact-sheets/ nfl-head-neck-and-spine-committee-s-concussion-diagnosis-and-management-protocol
6. Shea M. Forty Years of the Four Principles: Enduring Themes from Beauchamp and Childress. *The Journal of Medicine and Philosophy: A Forum for Bioethics and Philosophy of Medicine.* 2020;45(4–5):387–395. doi:10.1093/jmp/jhaa020
7. Beauchamp TL, Childress JF. *Principles of Biomedical Ethics.* 7th ed. Oxford University Press; 2013. https://utulsa.summon.serialssolutions.com/2.0.0/link/0/eLvH-CXMwY2AwNtIz0EUrE1KNLBINUxKTkpMSk1KSjMxSUhJTgFWVsQXoKMp Ec9C-YXc_EzdHI-cAExfosdvFiKEMvdKS0hzI3K4-fPTCyBS0ixNY_LIC-wgWFi wMrO7OzuEuiBEWc1NLYHqEnKNjCexnmFpYQo_cgfGBNQobxGikSsVNkIE FtNFAiIEpNU-YgcMXOsktwiAfABsAL1bIT1OAbJAHhaUC-K77YlEGeTfXEG cPXYiZ8dARmHiYU82NxBh4E0Er1_NKwDvcUiQYFBKBbRzjFGC3I9EkCTRJm-WRummRsZpxqam6QZJKUYizJIIHLOCncUtIMXEbgixtAgwUyDKxpwMScKgvzr-Rw0rACQj3KM
8. Sim J. Sports Medicine: Some Ethical Issues. *British Journal of Sports Medicine.* 1993;27(2):95–100.
9. *Dent v. National Football League*, No. 19-16017 (9th Cir. 2020). Justia Law. January 4, 2024. Accessed December 29, 2023. https://law.justia.com/cases/federal/ appellate-courts/ca9/19-16017/19-16017-2020-08-07.html
10. Spingola PM. Knapp v Northwestern University: The Seventh Circuit Slam Dunks the Rights of the Disabled. *Chi.-Kent L. Rev.* 1998; 73(3):709.
11. Orr RD, Pang N, Pellegrino ED, Siegler M. Use of the Hippocratic Oath: A Review of Twentieth Century Practice and a Content Analysis of Oaths Administered in Medical Schools in the U.S. and Canada in 1993. *The Journal of Clinical Ethics.* 1997;8(4):377–388. doi:10.1086/JCE199708409
12. nata_code_of_ethics_2022.pdf. Accessed March 18, 2023. https://www.nata.org/sites/ default/files/nata_code_of_ethics_2022.pdf
13. codeofethicshods06-20-28-25.pdf. Accessed March 18, 2023. https://www.apta.org/ siteassets/pdfs/policies/codeofethicshods06-20-28-25.pdf
14. Child Welfare Information Gateway. *Mandatory Reporters of Child Abuse and Neglect.* Updated 2023. Accessed November 1, 2024. https://www.childwelfare.gov/resources/ mandatory-reporting-child-abuse-and-neglect/
15. *McGowan v. S. Methodist Univ.*, Civil Action No. 3:18-CV-0141-N | Casetext Search + Citator. Accessed January 4, 2024. https://casetext.com/case/mcgowan-v-s-methodist-univ/
16. Civil Rights Division. *Title IX.* August 6, 2015. Accessed January 4, 2024. https://www. justice.gov/crt/title-ix

17. NCAA Basketball Player Calls Out Women's "Weight Room" in Viral TikTok. Accessed January 4, 2024. https://www.newsweek.com/ncaa-basketball-player-calls-out-womens-weight-room-viral-tiktok-1577401

18. ATRULES_09.2020.pdf.

19. Athletic Trainers Beware. *Training & Conditioning*. Accessed September 4, 2024. https://training-conditioning.com/article/athletic-trainers-beware/

20. Coach Makes the Call. *The Chronicle of Higher Education*. September 2, 2013. Accessed September 4, 2024. https://www.chronicle.com/article/coach-makes-the-call/

21. Are Billions of Dollars in Revenue Helping or Hurting College Sports? *Scripps News*. Accessed January 31, 2024. https://scrippsnews.com/stories/are-billions-of-dollars-in-revenue-helping-or-hurting-college-sports/

22. Rapp GC, Ingersoll CD. Sports Medicine Delivery Models: Legal Risks. *Journal of Athletic Training - Allen Press*. 2019;54(12):1237–1240.

4   Informed Consent

Chapter Objectives: Following the completion of this chapter, the reader will:

1. Define informed consent
2. Identify the components of informed consent
3. Lists the type of informed consent
4. Recognize and differentiate informed consent applied to various individuals
5. Apply examples of informed consent in clinical and research-based scenarios

Definition of Informed Consent

In the most simple explanation, the term "**informed consent**" can be summarized by a practitioner explaining to a patient an intervention to be performed in a way that the patient understands and agrees to having it done. Some say that this is characterized by having the practitioner act as a reasonable professional would act under similar circumstances. (Pachman) This would include providing the patient with sufficient relevant information about the associated risks and benefits of the proposed intervention in order for the patient to make an educated and autonomous decision about proceeding.[1]

The concept of informed consent was originally recognized by the US courts in the case Mohr v. Williams dating back to 1905. As one might expect, the initial concept of consent was to have in place a simple mechanism for a patient to provide consent for any medical treatment.[2] The term has evolved to mean a form of shorthand for all aspects of obtaining permission from a patient for a diagnostic or treatment intervention.[3]

Over the years, the term "doctrine of informed consent" has as "*a duty imposed by a healthcare provider to explain the risks associated with a recommended procedure prior to a patient determining whether or not to proceed the said procedure.*"[4]

From an athletic trainer's perspective, the process of informed consent carries both ethical and legal importance. An athletic trainer has an ethical responsibility to inform a patient of any associated risks and benefits of an intervention or technique, in addition to the mere fact that one is in fact qualified to perform said

DOI: 10.4324/9781003524823-4

activity. Legally, failure to obtain proper informed consent can be found to be a form of negligence and malpractice.

Required Components of Informed Consent

As the concept of providing informed consent has become more of an acceptable and required standard over time, more formal guidelines have been established to constitute the necessary components. As previously noted, the ultimate intent is for the provider of care to deliver the necessary information that a "reasonable person" would want to know prior to making an informed decision. In the absence of such information, it is fair to suggest that any decision made was not done so with the patient being appropriately informed. In addition to missing information, providing biased information may also constitute an unethical and potentially legal concern. In athletics, for example, influences exist from coaches and others that can lead to individuals not making decisions in their best interest.

While informed consent laws may vary slightly from state to state, in general, there will always be a shared responsibility between the athletic trainer and the patient as one is responsible for delivering as much information as necessary and the other must therefore make a decision based on what is provided. Given the same information provided, how the decisions made by patients may differ from one to another based upon their own personal circumstances.

There are four legal components that comprise required informed consent, these are as follows:

1. The patient is competent and of legal age.
2. A clear explanation of risks and benefits is provided.
3. The patient demonstrates an understanding of the information provided.
4. The patient's consent to consent is voluntary.

Let us look at each of these components individually. To begin with, anyone providing consent must be what the courts refer to as being competent. For an adult patient to be declared competent, certain criteria must exist[5] whereby a patient should:

- Be oriented to time, place, and person.
- Understand relevant information pertaining to the situation and proposed intervention.
- Clearly understand any benefits and risks associated with the situation and proposed interventions.
- Understand any consequences associated with available options, including opting not to participate or receive a proposed intervention.
- Clearly and voluntarily express consent absent any sign of coercion.

In the United States the legal age to provide informed consent is considered to be 18 years. With circumstances that are considered to be of moderate to high risk, a parent, guardian, or approved caregiver will be required to provide consent on behalf of a minor.[6]

(Salyanarayana) The exception to this could occur with a life or death or emergency situation whereby a treatment intervention may be required in a timely manner.

It is the responsibility of the athletic trainer and associated healthcare team to provide all necessary, adequate, and pertinent information to a patient or athlete regarding potential benefits and risks associated with a proposed intervention or decision. This also includes alternative options to proposed recommendations to ensure that an informed decision can be made. It is reasonable to assume that a vast amount of information must be disclosed to a patient to better formulate an informed decision. This may include, but is not limited to, providing a thorough explanation of one's condition and prognosis, proposed interventions and/or decisions to proceed with, associated benefits and risks, timelines for expected outcomes, and the opportunity to ask questions and receive accurate and timely responses. In truth, there is no set formula to determine how much information must be shared. However, at the end of the day there is a responsibility on the part of the athletic trainer to present all necessary information that would be deemed reasonable and prudent by an average person to need to know prior to making an informed decision.

An important component of informed consent is assurance that the patient clearly understands all of the information provided and disclosed by the athletic trainer. In addition to being thorough when conveying the information previously described, the method in which the information is shared is also of importance. The use of simple language in layperson terms, written drawings, anatomical models, and other visuals can be of help in explaining and further assuring one's understanding.

As has been previously mentioned, a patient's consent must be given voluntarily. This means that no undue outside influences, biases, or forms of coercion can be employed in an attempt to intentionally lead one's decision in a certain direction. Examples of this can come from coaches wanting an athlete to return to play despite further risk of a serious injury, parents having a personal opinion that possibly is different from the facts of the situation, and other individuals or circumstances that could cloud one's objective decision-making process. Confirmation of one's understanding is typically accomplished by way of a written signature. In some circumstances, a verbal confirmation can be accepted in the form of a positive response, such as a "yes" statement, or even a head nod in agreement. If anything greater than minimal risks are associated with one's decision, it is always best to obtain written consent. Technically speaking the consent is considered finalized with one's written signature. This serves as evidence that a conversation took place between the athletic trainer and the patient. However, it is important to recognize the role of shared decision-making and that what is most important is the actual conversation between the athletic trainer and the patient that leads to one's ultimate decision.

Types of Informed Consent

Written

It is commonly understood that a written form of consent is considered to be best practice for athletic trainers.[7] Since it is ultimately the responsibility of the athletic trainer to ensure that a patient comprehends and consents to a proposed intervention, having such verification in writing is always the best approach and is maintained as part of a medical record. Up to this point, the chapter discussed obtaining consent as it relates to a specific situation. At times, informed consent to participate in an activity in general is often obtained at the beginning of a sports season. Figure 4.1 provides an example of blanket informed consent in written format.

* Permission to reprint copyright 2025 Jeff G. Konin

Program/Activity Title:
[Insert Name of the Sport or Program]

Organization/Facility:
[Insert Organization Name and Address]

Date: [Insert Date]

---

1. Introduction and Purpose

You are invited to participate in [Sport/Program Name]. The purpose of this document is to provide you with clear and complete information about the nature of the sport activity, including its potential risks and benefits, so that you can make an informed decision about your participation. Your involvement is entirely voluntary.

---

2. Description of the Sport Activity

- **Activity Overview:**
  [Describe the sport, training sessions, competitions, or recreational activities involved.]
- **Duration and Schedule:**
  [Outline the expected duration, session frequency, and any seasonal or event-specific details.]
- **Location:**
  [Provide details about where the sport activities will take place.]

Figure 4.1 Example of a blanket written informed consent

3. Risks and Discomforts

Participation in sports involves inherent risks. Please review the following potential risks and acknowledge your understanding:

- **Physical Injuries:**
  You may experience injuries such as sprains, strains, fractures, concussions, or other physical impacts.
- **Environmental Risks:**
  Risks related to weather conditions, playing surfaces, equipment malfunction, or unforeseen accidents.
- **Other Potential Discomforts:**
  Fatigue, muscle soreness, or other temporary discomforts associated with physical exertion.

While every effort is made to ensure a safe environment, no activity is without risk. It is important that you understand and accept these risks before participating.

---

4. Benefits of Participation

Participation in [Sport/Program Name] may offer several benefits, including:

- Improved physical fitness and overall health.
- Enhanced skills, teamwork, and discipline.
- Opportunities for personal growth, social interaction, and community engagement.
- Enjoyment and recreational satisfaction.

---

5. Confidentiality and Data Protection

Any personal information collected during your participation will be kept confidential and used solely for program-related purposes, including performance monitoring and safety procedures. Data will be stored securely, and your identity will not be disclosed in any public reports without your consent.

---

6. Voluntary Participation and Right to Withdraw

- **Voluntary Participation:**
  Your participation in this sport is completely voluntary. You have the right to decide not to participate or to withdraw from the activity at any time without penalty.
- **Right to Withdraw:**
  If you choose to withdraw, please notify [Program Coordinator/Instructor's Name] at [Contact Information]. Your decision to withdraw will not affect your relationship with the organization or any future opportunities.

Figure 4.1 (Continued)

7. Emergency Medical Treatment

In the event of an injury or medical emergency during participation, you authorize the staff to provide first aid or emergency medical treatment. You understand that every effort will be made to contact you or your emergency contact as soon as possible.

Emergency Contact Information:

- Name: _____
- Phone Number: _____

8. Consent Statement

By signing below, you acknowledge that:

- You have read and understood the information provided in this document.
- You are aware of the potential risks and benefits associated with participating in [Sport/Program Name].
- Your participation is voluntary, and you have had the opportunity to ask questions.
- You agree to abide by all rules, instructions, and safety guidelines established by the organization.

Participant's Name (Printed): _____

Participant's Signature: _____

Date: _____

If the participant is a minor (under 18 years of age), parental or guardian consent is required.

Parent/Guardian Name (Printed): _____

Parent/Guardian Signature: _____

Date: _____

Disclaimer: This is a basic informed consent template for sports participation. It is intended to serve as a guide and should be modified to meet the specific needs and legal requirements of your organization and the sport activity in question. Top of FormBottom of Form

Figure 4.1 (Continued)

Verbal

Under some circumstances, a verbal consent process may be appropriate. Verbal consent is where a patient states their consent to a procedure verbally through voice affirmation or clear body language but does not sign any written form. Whenever verbal consent is utilized, it is recommended that, at minimum, the following information is obtained:

- Name of the patient providing verbal consent (Or adult if for a minor)
- Name of the person obtaining verbal consent
- Date and time of verbal consent
- Method by which verbal consent is obtained (phone, video call, in person)
- Name of a witness to the verbal consent
- A succinct, accurate summary of consenting facts

Additional Considerations for Obtaining Informed Consent

There are some additional considerations for obtaining informed consent under special circumstances. One example is that of when treating a patient who is pregnant. During pregnancy, informed consent can be described as the process of decision-making between a patient and the healthcare provider regarding the clinical management of the pregnancy. Given the nature of the sensitivity of bodily changes and decision-making for more than one individual, additional care must be taken to ensure that appropriate information is shared. Primarily, information shared must also include all of the risks associated with not only the individual patient who is childbearing but also those associated with the child for both current and future considerations.

Prisoners have been recognized as a class of individuals who require special attention due to their circumstances. In many cases, these concerns relate to research methods where the risks involved in research studies that prisoners take part in must be commensurate with risks that would be accepted by a non-prisoner participant. Once again, given the environment that prisoners live in, additional considerations of fairness, equity, and specifically that no future bias toward an individual will be displayed by not voluntarily participating in a research study.

A type of research study that requires informed consent but in its own unique way does not intentionally provide all of the facts to a volunteering participant is referred to as deception. Deception occurs when a researcher provides less than honest information to a study participant or intentionally misleads them about a part of the study. Why then would someone consent to participate in a study where known deception is occurring? A deceptive study is performed as a means of not having participants influence their own results. A simple example unrelated to healthcare is when participants may be asked to give a speech, and they are told the speech will be recorded. Informed consent may include measuring one's level of stress in particular as it is related to knowingly being recorded. In fact, the speeches may not be recorded and the investigators may be measuring one stress level solely on the perception of one's anxiety for being recorded. In medical research, a placebo intervention is oftentimes used, and it is compared to real interventions in an effort to compare outcomes. If subjects' consent to knowing one of the possible trials of the study will include a placebo intervention, this is not deception. However, if subjects are told that all of the possible trials will include some form of an actual treatment intervention, and one in fact does not, this would constitute deception. This would be done for the purposes of identifying subjects' perceptive responses under the impression of having a real treatment intervention.

Practical Examples of Informed Consent

Circumstances that require informed consent can be found in every setting that an athletic trainer may be employed. In an athletic training clinic, the delivery of therapeutic ultrasound is not uncommon as a form of treatment intervention. As a patient, perhaps you have never seen ultrasound used before, let alone on you. Imagine someone waving some kind of a wand your way that is plugged into a wall and headed your way! What will it feel like? Is it supposed to be uncomfortable? Warm? Cold? How long will this last? Will I feel any different after it is completed? If so, when, and for how long? To the patient who has no understanding from either a scientific or layperson viewpoint, all aspects of the use of the ultrasound treatment should be explained clearly and in a manner that is understood prior to obtaining the patient's informed consent to proceed. How will you explain the transference of electrical energy to acoustical energy? Does the patient need to know this is called a reverse piezoelectric effect? If you describe what is happening in terms of "sound waves," might that make a patient nervous or apprehensive? After all, how often in life does someone apply sound waves to you? As an athletic trainer, you should not only have this information in written form to obtain a patient's consent, but you should also have a well-rehearsed explanation of ultrasound delivery and be prepared to honestly answer any questions. Adding a medication such as a topical hydrocortisone adds an additional dimension to information sharing. Take a moment to reflect on how you would actually convey this verbally prior to reading on. When you are around others, try your explanation out on them and gather feedback to fine-tune your delivery of information.

Another very common and slightly more complicated informed consent that is required would be that of a return to play from an injury. We simply refer to this as "return to play" or "RTP." When providing a patient/player/athlete with the necessary information prior to making a decision of whether or not one is "ready" to return to play in a competitive environment, a thorough consideration of the benefits and the potential risks must be included. It is the responsibility of the athletic trainer to inform one of any risk of further injury, more severe injury, as well as additional potential complications both short and long terms. The actual return-to-play decision is oftentimes not the difficult part of a situation. Discussing the decision with the athlete may well be the bigger challenge. The conversation itself is, ideally, conducted in an office or athletic training clinic without where there is no overbearing sense of time constraint or pressure to make a quick decision. Compare this to the sidelines of a sporting event with the game on the line, the adrenaline of the moment, and others surrounding you within very close proximity adding to the pressures of the exchange itself. Furthermore, one may literally have seconds to provide the information with more than likely less than optimal time for one to weigh the options and take into account the full risks versus benefits. In sideline situations such as this, the athletic trainer is not exempt from delivering the same level of information, and must also follow through with documentation to support the exchange and ultimate decision. This is a less-than-desirable atmosphere for legal purposes of meeting the standards of informed consent. However, this is a reality that all athletic trainers face very often. Therefore, a well-thought-out plan to deliver comprehensive and accurate information in an expedited manner should be inclusive of one's strategy. Furthermore, collaboration and communication with colleagues can be helpful in establishing a process that would comply with the law as best as possible in terms of doing what a reasonable and prudent athletic trainer would do under the same circumstances. Keep in mind, despite a well-implemented plan, a resultant injury can still put an athletic trainer at legal risk for negligence partially based upon how the sideline informed consent process was carried out.

In a landmark case, Kruger v. San Francisco 49ers[8], the First US Court of Appeals determined that the Forty-Niners team physicians did not fully disclose the potential adverse effects resulting from ongoing steroid injections into Mr. Kruger's knee during the season. The team and physicians were held liable because they failed to make full disclosers on the potential long-term effects of participating with a significant knee injury.

Another consideration of informed consent relates to practitioner disclosure of information. That is, does the individual providing services have an obligation to reveal any personal medical history that could impact the care or intervention being provided? While rare, anyone providing care that is in a position to transmit any adverse conditions to others may fall under such circumstances. This so-called duty to inform has recently been brought to light as a result of the SARS Covid-19 virus where individuals provide care to others could potentially be infected and/or a carrier of the virus.[3]

Undue Influence

Undue influence has been mentioned previously because it can place added pressure to reach a decision following informed consent particularly as it relates to return-to-play scenarios. For example, during a game when a player is injured, the athletic trainer has the responsibility of assessing whether or not it is safe for the player to return to competition. The player should be made aware of any risk associated with returning to play and being a part of the decision to return or not. Consider a scenario where one encounters a minor knee ligament injury, any associated risk for returning to play could include further damage to the knee ligaments as well as other bodily injury as a result of participating with functional deficits. Again, it is the athletic trainer's responsibility to convey all relevant information. With the risk of returning to play accurately conveyed to the participant, the individual must willingly agree to want to return to play on one's own volition. In a relatively all too common scenario, outside pressures exerted by coaches, parents, and others can provide undue influence on one's decision-making process and unnecessarily place an individual in harm's way. Coaches may consider this to be a key player who in their mind is "better at 75%" as compared to the backup player who would fill the role. This is coach thinking but should not be a part of the athletic trainer's discussion. Furthermore, parents may be caught up in the chain of events especially if their son or daughter is a senior in high school and there are college coaches scouting him/her for a potential scholarship. Is the child tough enough to battle, will he/she lose a scholarship if injured and not playing? Will game statistics be impacted? These are all examples of what we call undo influences that can cloud the decision-making of a return-to-play scenario. While the athletic trainer should remain cognizant of their presence, these should not factor into the medical benefits and risks.

Emergent Situations

In an emergent situation informed consent is not required to be obtained. With emergencies, a patient's health or safety may be at risk if treatment is delayed because consent cannot be obtained as may be seen when an athlete on a field becomes unconscious and unable to comprehend and respond. Informed consent is also not required in a circumstance where the parents of a seriously ill or injured minor cannot be reached. Even in emergency situations, medical personnel are generally allowed to only administer the level of treatment that is necessary to stabilize a patient until proper consent can be obtained.

Informed Consent in Research

When individuals, otherwise referred to as "human subjects," are sought to participate in a research study, all of the details of the study are required to be shared with the potential participant in layperson terms so that one can voluntarily participate with the full knowledge of the study's purpose, methods and procedures, risks, and benefits. Figure 4.2 outlines components of information that should be included in an informed consent discussion for research while Figure 4.3 provides an example of a general written document for consent to participate in a research study.

Such forms that include minors are designed to have adult and/or parental/guardian approval.

1. **Introduction and Purpose**
   - Explain the purpose of the procedure, treatment, or study in clear, accessible language.
2. **Description of Procedures**
   - Outline what will happen during the procedure or study, including steps, timeline, and any specific activities involved.
3. **Potential Risks and Discomforts**
   - Detail possible risks, side effects, or discomforts that might be experienced, ensuring that patients understand what could go wrong.
4. **Potential Benefits**
   - Explain the possible benefits, both direct (to the patient) and indirect (to future patients or scientific knowledge).
5. **Alternatives**
   - Describe available alternatives, including the option not to participate or receive the procedure, along with the associated implications.
6. **Confidentiality and Data Handling**
   - Provide information on how the patient's personal and medical information will be protected, stored, and possibly used in future research or reports.
7. **Voluntary Participation and Right to Withdraw**
   - Emphasize that participation is completely voluntary and that the patient can withdraw at any time without affecting their care or services.
8. **Compensation and Costs**
   - If applicable, explain any compensation for participation and detail any costs that the patient might incur.
9. **Contact Information for Questions or Concerns**
   - List contact details for the principal investigator or designated staff, and provide information on whom to contact if any concerns arise (e.g., an ethics committee or review board).
10. **Consent Statement and Signatures**
    - Include a clear statement confirming that the patient understands the information and agrees to participate.
    - Provide space for the patient's signature, the date, and, if needed, a witness's signature.

Figure 4.2 Components of information that should be included in an informed consent document for research

Informed Consent Document

Title of Study:
[Insert Study Title]

Principal Investigator:
[Name, Title] [Department, Institution] [Contact Information]

IRB Protocol Number:
[Insert Protocol Number]

Version & Date:
[Version Number, Date]

---

1. Introduction

You are invited to participate in a research study conducted by [Principal Investigator's Name]. Before you decide to participate, please read the following information carefully. This document explains the purpose of the study, the procedures involved, and your rights as a participant. Your participation is entirely voluntary.

---

2. Purpose of the Study

The purpose of this study is to: [Provide a brief description of the study objectives and why it is being conducted.]

---

3. Study Procedures

If you agree to participate, you will be asked to:

- [Describe what participants will do, e.g., complete questionnaires, undergo interviews, etc.]
- [State the duration of participation and the frequency of procedures.]

Location of the study: [Provide location details, if applicable.]

Figure 4.3 Example of an informed consent document for human research

4. Risks and Discomforts

Participation in this study may involve risks and discomforts, including:

- [Describe any physical, emotional, or psychological risks.]
- [Explain any procedures that might cause discomfort.]

Every precaution will be taken to minimize these risks. Should any unexpected issues arise, they will be addressed promptly.

5. Potential Benefits

While there is no guarantee that you will directly benefit from participating, this study may help to:

- [Describe potential benefits, such as contributing to scientific knowledge or improving practices.]

Your participation may also benefit others in the future by providing valuable information for [research, treatment, policy, etc.].

6. Confidentiality

The information you provide will be kept confidential and stored securely. Measures to protect your data include:

- [Describe data storage, access controls, and de-identification procedures.]
- Your identity will not be disclosed in any reports or publications resulting from this study, except as required by law.

7. Voluntary Participation and Withdrawal

- **Voluntary Participation:** Your decision to participate is completely voluntary.
- **Right to Withdraw:** You may decline to participate or withdraw from the study at any time without penalty or loss of benefits to which you are otherwise entitled.
- **No Impact on Services:** Withdrawing from the study will not affect your current or future relationship with [Institution or Service Provider].

Figure 4.3 (Continued)

8. Compensation (if applicable)

- [Detail any compensation provided for participation or explain that there is no compensation.]

9. Questions and Contact Information

If you have any questions about this study or your rights as a research participant, please contact:
Principal Investigator: [Name] [Phone Number] [Email Address]
If you have questions about your rights or feel you have been treated unfairly, you may contact the Institutional Review Board at: [IRB Contact Information]

10. Consent Statement

By signing below, you acknowledge that you have read and understood the information provided above, and you voluntarily agree to participate in this study. You will receive a copy of this document for your records.

Participant's Printed Name: _____

Participant's Signature: _____ **Date:** _____

Investigator's Signature: _____ **Date:** _____

Disclaimer: This is a basic informed consent template and may require modifications to meet the specific needs of your study and comply with all relevant institutional and regulatory requirements.
Bottom of Form

Figure 4.3 (Continued)

Summary

It is the responsibility of the athletic trainer to meet the standard of care with respect to informed consent. If not, one can be held legally responsible for future injuries that may occur in the absence of full disclosure of the risks by the athletic trainer to the patient.

Informed consent is a relatively new phenomenon. Its requirements unsurprisingly evolve as societal values and expectations change. Patient autonomy in clinical decision-making is now paramount. The underlying assumption for IC doctrine is that the physician's basic thinking be transparent to the patient to provide valid care.

This necessitates more than simply explaining the risks and benefits of any proposed care. The physician must explain their decision-making process. This transparency relates to the disclosure of all matters, medical and non-medical, that may influence the HCP's delivery of that care and affect the patient's informed decision.

References

1. *Sports Medicine Legal Digest.* 1:1. Accessed October 16, 2024. https://pubs.royle.com/publication/?i=408268&view=archiveBrowser
2. Bunch WH, Dvonch VM. Informed Consent in Sports Medicine. *Clinics in Sports Medicine.* 2004;23(2):183–193. doi:10.1016/j.csm.2004.01.004
3. Simpson JK, Innes S. Informed Consent, Duty of Disclosure and Chiropractic: Where Are We? *Chiropractic & Manual Therapies.* 2020;28(1):2–12, 60. doi:10.1186/s12998-020-00342-5
4. Mallardi V. Le Origini del Consenso Informato [The Origin of Informed Consent]. *Acta Otorhinolaryngologica Italica.* 2005;25(5):312–327.
5. Shea M. Forty Years of the Four Principles: Enduring Themes from Beauchamp and Childress. *The Journal of Medicine and Philosophy: A Forum for Bioethics and Philosophy of Medicine.* 2020;45(4–5):387–395. doi:10.1093/jmp/jhaa020
6. Rao KHS. Informed Consent: An Ethical Obligation or Legal Compulsion? *Journal of Cutaneous and Aesthetic Surgery.* 2008;1(1):33–35. doi:10.4103/0974-2077.41159
7. best-practice-guidelines-for-athletic-training-documentation.pdf. Accessed October 16, 2024. https://www.nata.org/sites/default/files/best-practice-guidelines-for-athletic-training-documentation.pdf
8. *Krueger v. San Franscico Forty Niners and Epstein v. Enterprise Leasing Corp.,* Justia Law. October 23, 2024. Accessed October 16, 2024. https://law.justia.com/cases/california/court-of-appeal/3d/189/823.html

5 Standard of Care

Chapter Objectives: Following the completion of this chapter, the reader will:

1. Apply the concept of standard of care to the relevant areas of clinical practice.
2. Recognize the role position and consensus statements play in establishing standards of care.
3. Analyze the relationship between standards of care and evidence-based practice.

As presented in Chapter 1, negligence exists only when the four elements of negligence, duty, breach, cause, and harm are present. In essence, the defendant must owe a duty to the plaintiff and a subsequent breach of that duty did, in fact, cause some harm or damage to the plaintiff.[1] In most cases involving physicians[2] or other clinicians, the issue of duty is both readily apparent and legally sound. The existence of a clinician–patient relationship implies the provider of services, in this case, the clinician, has a duty to the patient. Henry Terry[3] stated very simply but accurately that negligence exists when one fails to act as a reasonable and prudent person. Determining what is reasonable and prudent, or what was or was not a breach of duty, can become complicated when the actor under scrutiny is a healthcare professional. Medical malpractice dates to the year 1374 in England.[4] In that instance, a physician was sued over alleged improper management of a patient with a hand injury, but it was not until the middle of the 19th century that medical care providers were commonly expected to deliver services that were, obviously, very different from the capabilities of the average citizen.

As the practice of medicine evolved, so did expectations for the level of care provided by the physician. Gradually, as medicine and healthcare evolved, the concept of standard of care began to take shape. As medical providers became better qualified, the expectations placed upon them by their patients advanced as well. Technically speaking, the standard of care is defined as treatment that is "accepted by medical experts as a proper treatment for a certain type of disease that is widely used by healthcare professionals."[5] Failure to provide that standard of care qualifies as the breach element of negligence. The challenge lies in identifying the standard of care that is appropriate. There are many factors, or doctrines, that influence the appropriate standard of care, some of which are unique in that they exist solely in

DOI: 10.4324/9781003524823-5

association with medical care.[4] The locality rule is one of the oldest of those doctrines which can complicate the issue of the standard of care as it has been in existence since 1880.[6] The locality rule dictates that the actions of a physician must be evaluated and compared to the actions of physicians within the same geographical region or locality. For example, the actions of a physician in Florida could not be accurately compared to those of a physician in California. The concept of "locality" being a major element of standard of care seems difficult to imagine, and yet, Ginsburg[7] voiced strong opposition to the application of the doctrine as recently as 2012. It is not suggested that a "locality rule" exists for athletic trainers. The fact remains, however, that identifying a standard of care is not always entirely straightforward.

Standard of Care

During a September 15, 1995, football game between Cedar Bluff High School and Beemer High School, Brent Cerny suffered a head injury. There were no athletic trainers present during the game and the injury was managed by the coaches for Cedar Bluff High School.[7] After the injury it is agreed that Cerny was slightly symptomatic, more specifically that he was having difficulty catching his breath, but Cedar Bluffs coaches believed Cerny was hyperventilating and showed no other signs related to a head injury. Both coaches reported Cerny responded normally and made good eye contact when questioned. Cerny re-entered play later in the game and was reported by both coaches to be normal. Cerny later testified that he had a persistent headache from the time of injury until the next practice on Tuesday. There is no clear evidence that Cerny reported his headache to either coach. Physicians later testified that in their opinion Cerny suffered from second impact syndrome when he returned to practice while still having symptoms of a head injury, leaving him with permanent brain damage.

Whether the coaches owed a duty to Cerny was never an issue. The issue was, however, what standard of care was expected as the coaches fulfilled their duty to provide care for the injured player. Standard of care can be defined as the degree of care a person is expected to provide and is based on that person's level of training and expected expertise.[5] Obviously, neither coach had extensive medical training and was not expected to function at the level of an emergency physician. However, both did have the minimal level of training needed to obtain a coaching certificate in the state of Nebraska. Experts testified that this level of training included a basic course in the prevention and treatment of athletic injuries. It was determined that both coaches could reasonably be expected to know the signs and symptoms of a concussion as well as knowing not to allow the injured athlete to return to play while symptomatic.[7]

The standard of care expected from individuals can vary greatly and depends on exactly who is providing the care. In the Cerny case, an emergency room physician would certainly have been held to a higher standard. Had the coaches not been required to complete the prevention and treatment course to obtain their state coaching certificate, they would likely have been held to a lower standard.

It becomes immediately apparent that the specific level of education required of an individual is a key influence on expected standards of behavior. Educational background is one influence but there are many others that are examined in the remainder of this chapter.

Many professional associations publish[8–10] position statements or consensus statements relative to specific issues that impact the practice of members of that association. The National Athletic Trainers' Association (NATA) is certainly an example of that as it publishes a number of different types of statements that can factor into identifying standards of practice, or standards of care, for athletic trainers. The NATA partners with the NATA Research and Education Foundation (Foundation) to develop and publish position statements, official statements, consensus statements, and support statements. Of primary importance are position statements, which represent the official opinion of the association on a given situation or scenario. Position statements are developed by a team of athletic trainers with expertise specific to the area and represent a substantial scholarly effort. Consensus statements represent the agreement of several associations or agencies like the NATA that have expertise and are involved in the topic under discussion.

The "Consensus Recommendations on the Prehospital Care of the Injured Athlete With a Suspected Catastrophic Cervical Injury"[10] is a good example of a position statement developed by multiple agencies working cooperatively. The statement was developed by athletic trainers, emergency room physicians, orthopedic surgeons, emergency medical technicians, and researchers after extensive examination of existing literature and policy. The result is an organized and reliable review of over 1,500 studies related to the topic. The statement represents the agreement of those individuals and in essence, the groups they represent. Official statements are also published by the NATA and typically address topics or issues that are very time sensitive.

Position statements are credible, reliable resources to use in identifying acceptable standards of care. Consider that in the previously mentioned consensus statement on pre-hospital care of the cervical spine-injured athlete, the process included a systematic review comprised of 1,544 studies, 49 of which were included in the final full-text review. Using the results of the systematic review as a shared evidence base, the nominal group technique meeting created and refined conclusions and recommendations until consensus was achieved.

While based on credible research, official statements are briefer than a position or consensus statement and represent only the position taken specifically by the NATA. The NATA also publishes Support Statements which document the endorsement or support of a NATA initiative or practice by another group of professionals. One such example is the American Academy of Family Physicians' support statement for placing athletic trainers in secondary schools[11].

Evidence-Based Medicine and the Standard of Care

Athletic trainers practicing in the USA must adhere to, among other things, the code of conduct outlined by the credentialing agency, the Board of Certification,

Inc. (BOC).[12] The BOC Standards for Professional Practice includes two sections. The first section presents practice standards, and the second section includes codes for professional responsibility. Within the Code of Professional Responsibility, it is specifically stated that athletic trainers must "demonstrate sound clinical judgement that is based upon current knowledge, evidence-based guidelines and the thoughtful and safe application of resources." Evidence-based practice is not a new concept for healthcare providers. Students in education programs in athletic training are taught how to read and critique research in an effort to make them responsible consumers of new knowledge that will influence their clinical decision-making process. It would seem at first glance that a push toward new or current knowledge diminishes the importance of established standards of practice. At first glance that might seem logical, however, there is an abundance of case law[13] that supports athletic trainers following recognized standards of care as established by learned bodies in athletic training and substantiated by research. The challenge for athletic trainers, or any healthcare provider, in maintaining clinical competency, is to consider both established standards and current research and new knowledge[14]. Courts have long recognized the duty of a healthcare provider to remain knowledgeable about the most current research and techniques. In fact, numerous medical texts were cited as evidence in an early case that dates back to 1850[15]. In doing so the court clearly acknowledged that a trained physician should have a certain level of knowledge that is included in the standard medical school curriculum. In the same case, the court also stated a trained physician is expected to use their best clinical judgment in combination with those established practice standards.

For athletic trainers, the primary source of practice standards is the[16] National Athletic Trainers' Association Research and Education Foundation (Foundation). The Foundation works with the National Athletic Trainers' Association (NATA) in overseeing the development and dissemination of position statements and consensus statements that function as practice standards for the profession. The NATA and the Foundation have cooperatively published over two dozen position statements that help guide clinical decision-making and practice in athletic training. Both the NATA and the Foundation include verbiage accompanying those position statements emphatically stating the documents are not be-all, end-all substitutes for professional judgment as influenced by specific circumstances or laws.

"The NATA publishes its position statements as a service to promote the awareness of certain issues to its members. The information contained in the position statement is neither exhaustive nor exclusive to all circumstances or individuals. Variables, such as institutional human resource guidelines, state or federal statutes, rules, or regulations, as well as regional environmental conditions, may impact the relevance and implementation of these recommendations. The NATA advises its members and others to carefully and independently consider each of the recommendations (including the applicability of same to any particular circumstance or individual). The position statement should not be relied upon as an independent basis for care, but rather as a resource available to NATA members or others. Moreover, no opinion is expressed herein regarding the quality of care that adheres to or differs from NATA's position statements. The NATA reserves the right to rescind or modify its position statements at any time."[16]

Taken directly from the NATA Research and Education Foundation website

References

1. Owen DG. The Five Elements of Negligence Idea. *Hofstra Law Review*. 2006;35(4): 1671–1686.
2. McCoid AH. The Care Required of Medical Practitioners. *Vanderbilt Law Review*. 1959;12:85.
3. Terry HT. Negligence. *Harvard Law Review*. 1915;29(1):40–54. doi:10.2307/1325735
4. Silver T. One Hundred Years of Harmful Error: The Historical Jurisprudence of Medical Malpractice. *Wisconsin Law Review*. 51.
5. How Standard of Care Depends on the Circumstances. *The Law Dictionary*. Accessed September 29, 2021. https://thelawdictionary.org/article/standard-of-care/
6. 128 Mass. 131 (Mass. 1880), Small v. Howard. *vLex*. Accessed March 14, 2022. https://case-law.vlex.com/vid/128-mass-131-mass-615569126
7. *Cerny v Cedar Bluffs Junior/Senior Public Schools*. N.W. 2d 628, 697
8. AOTA Official Documents. *AOTA*. Accessed September 11, 2022. https://www.aota.org/practice/practice-essentials/aota-official-documents
9. APTA Position Papers. *APTA*. Accessed September 11, 2022. https://www.apta.org/advocacy/position-papers
10. Mills BM, Conrick KM, Anderson S, et al. Consensus Recommendations on the Prehospital Care of the Injured Athlete with a Suspected Catastrophic Cervical Spine Injury. *Journal of Athletic Training*. 2020;55(6):563–572. doi:10.4085/1062-6050-0434.19
11. *Athletic Trainers for High School Athletes*. Accessed March 15, 2022. https://www.aafp.org/about/policies/all/athletic-trainers-high-school-athletes.html
12. 2021-BOC-Standards-of-Professional-Practice-Published-11-20-2020.pdf. Accessed September 9, 2022. https://nau.edu/wp-content/uploads/sites/167/2021-BOC-Standards-of-Professional-Practice-Published-11-20-2020.pdf
13. Anderson B, Parr A. Risk Management: Determining The Standard of Care. *Athletic Therapy Today*. 2006;11(1):6–68. doi:10.1123/att.11.1.6
14. Williams CL. Evidence-Based Medicine in the Law Beyond Clinical Practice Guidelines: What Effect Will EBM Have on the Standard of Care? *Washington and Lee Law Review*. 2011;61:479. https://scholarlycommons.law.wlu.edu/wlulr/vol61/iss1/10
15. *McCandless v. McWha*, 22 Pa. 261 (1853) | Caselaw Access Project. Accessed September 11, 2022. https://cite.case.law/pa/22/261/
16. *Position Statements—NATA Research & Education Foundation*. Accessed September 11, 2022. https://www.natafoundation.org/at-profession/position-statements/

6   Documentation in Athletic Training

Upon completion of this chapter, the reader will be able to:

1. Explain the importance of documentation in athletic training.
2. Identify and describe the types of documentation used in education and clinical practice.
3. Apply best practice strategies for effective documentation.

Introduction

In healthcare, documentation is a cornerstone of professional practice that serves as a safeguard for both the patient and the provider. Foundational concepts and principles of documentation are taught and assessed in accredited athletic training programs through varied methods, including the utilization of comprehensive patient-file management systems to document patient encounters, performing administrative duties related to athletic training, and the implementation of quality assurance and quality improvement measures to improve patient care[1]. Upon entering the workforce, credentialed athletic trainers are expected to utilize standard documentation procedures as outlined in the 8th edition of the Board of Certification (BOC) Practice Analysis[2] and ensuring confidentiality as outlined in the BOC Standards of Professional Practice[3].

As documentation practices have evolved from handwritten notes to the use of electronic health records that can be accessed by multiple providers, it is critical that healthcare providers engage in sound documentation practices. Clear, concise, accurate, and timely documentation of patient encounters can be an effective risk management strategy and can decrease the chances of medical error[4,5]. In 2017, the National Athletic Trainers' Association (NATA) published the "Best Practices Guidelines for Athletic Training Documentation"[6] which outlines strategies for implementing documentation practices that are in alignment with established best practices. Additionally, while the onus is on the provider, patients can play an active role in decreasing the chances of error by confirming their understanding of the procedure, asking about unfamiliar or unplanned tests, and verifying the information recorded is accurate[7].

DOI: 10.4324/9781003524823-6

As such, the purpose of this chapter is to highlight several of the key documents that athletic trainers should utilize, discuss best practices for documentation, and highlight why documentation is an effective risk management strategy.

Documentation in Athletic Training Education

Before diving into documentation specifically geared toward clinical practice, it is important to briefly highlight the importance of documentation in an educational program or academic setting. Professional, or entry-level, accredited academic programs are governed by the 2020 Commission on Accreditation of Athletic Training Education (CAATE) Standards[1], whereas accredited residencies and fellowships are governed by the 2022 CAATE Standards[8]. Programs must demonstrate compliance with each of the standards and provide evidence of how these standards are being addressed and assessed throughout the curriculum. To maintain accreditation, programs must submit an annual report to demonstrate how they are meeting the minimum compliance standards during the years when they do not undergo a peer-reviewed site visit[1, 8]. Additionally, educational programs must maintain student records related to student outcome measures, programmatic outcomes, affiliation agreements with clinical sites, the pass rate on the BOC certification examination, job placements, academic progress and advising, and academic misconduct[3, 8]. Institutions may also require additional specific reports to maintain compliance with overall university accreditation standards. This type of documentation is crucial for monitoring student development and progress, ensuring compliance with accreditation standards, and maintaining detailed records of clinical and educational experiences. Furthermore, it fosters and supports effective communication between students, professors, preceptors, and administrators to ensure accountability and continuous improvement of the educational experience.

Types of Documentation in Athletic Training Clinical Practice

Athletic trainers rely on a variety of documents to reflect the comprehensive and patient-centered care provided, with each document outlined subsequently serving a unique purpose. From injury reports to emergency action plans and insurance claims to rehabilitation plans, the depth and breadth of documentation that athletic trainers need to keep up with is essential in ensuring the patient's safety and well-being. As such, the remainder of this chapter focuses on the major categories of documentation that clinical athletic trainers should be utilizing in their own professional practice. Of note, the list subsequently is a representation of the types of documents athletic trainers should keep and is not an all-encompassing list. It is important to defer to institutional policies and procedures for additional documents that may be required.

Clinical Notes: One of the most important documents that athletic trainers keep are clinic notes, or SOAP notes. The acronym SOAP (subjective, objective, assessment, plan) provides a structured methodology for athletic trainers to follow as they are evaluating or re-evaluating a patient[9]. These notes should be detailed and reflective of the clinical examination performed by the athletic trainer or healthcare provider. The SOAP note structure can be used for a multitude of patient encounters to include initial evaluation, follow-up visits, and discharge notes. Furthermore, these notes are helpful with monitoring patient progression or identifying the onset and progression of injuries and illnesses.

Daily Sign-In Logs: This document is an account of the patient volume in the athletic training facility on a given day and can be organized to identify services provided (i.e., preventative, rehabilitative, evaluative). Furthermore, the data from these logs can be extrapolated to provide information on peak facility usage times, types of services being utilized, and an accountability tool to help with patient compliance and continuity of care.

Injury Reports: This document provides an account of the injury status of patients that can be shared with key stakeholders such as coaches. These reports provide status updates on injured players, approximately return-to-play timelines, and any other pertinent updates (i.e., upcoming surgical dates, scheduled doctors' visits, and rehabilitation highlights) that may be helpful to coaches and other stakeholders.

Treatment/Rehabilitation Plans: This document provides an account of all treatment and rehabilitation exercises the patient performed each day. The athletic trainer can use these documents to track a patient's progress through their injury, record any setbacks or deviations from the treatment protocol, and set goals for future recovery milestones.

Patient-Rated Outcome Measures (PROMs): These questionnaires can be helpful to athletic trainers to assess the impact of a patient's injury or illness on their overall health and quality of life. These measures often go beyond the impact of the injury on sports performance and address qualities such as the impact on daily activities of living, mental well-being, and functional ability. These tools are validated and reliable and can be used repeatedly throughout a patient's injury or illness.

Medical Referral Forms: These documents are used to help facilitate communication between the athletic trainer and external healthcare providers. Pertinent patient medical history, current treatment and condition updates, and the reason for the referral are clearly articulated on the form and provide useful information for the external provider.

Insurance Documents: Accurate and up-to-date insurance information is an essential part of the administrative work of an athletic trainer. Primary insurance information and copies of insurance cards should be collected as part of the pre-participation paperwork and updated annually. Additionally, it is important to remind patients to update their information if insurance information changes during the year. Furthermore, it is important that athletic trainers have an awareness of the types of insurance their patients hold and what restrictions or additional steps need to be taken for external care (i.e., referral from primary care doctor and in-network vs. out-of-network coverage)

Inventory Reports: Athletic trainers should maintain an up-to-date and accurate inventory of all supplies and equipment in the athletic training facility. This document allows athletic trainers to have a better understanding of how expendable items (i.e., tape), non-expendable items (i.e., braces), and capital equipment (i.e., modality units) are being utilized and maintained in the facility. This information can help athletic trainers decide which items and how much to purchase each year, as well as identify items that need to be repaired or replaced.

Emergency Action Plans (EAP): An emergency action plan (EAP) is defined as "a document detailing the preparation and on-site emergency response of health care professionals and other stakeholders to medical emergencies in the pre-hospital setting"[10]. In 2024, the NATA published an updated position statement titled "Emergency Action Plan Development and Implementation in Sport"[10] which provides comprehensive, detailed, and evidence-based strategies for the development and implementation of EAPs in clinical practice. Additional information about EAPs can be found in Chapter 2 of this textbook.

Policy & Procedure Manuals: These manuals outline the daily operating procedures within an athletic training facility. Many of the documents outlined earlier can be found in the policy and procedure manual for the facility, in addition to items such as staff duties and responsibilities. This manual, which should be reviewed and updated annually, can be helpful to ensure consistent delivery of care.

Continuing Education Requirements: Every two years, athletic trainers must submit the requisite documentation to the BOC for maintenance of their certification. Detailed information about these requirements can be found on the BOC website[11], which are regularly updated. The BOC periodically audits these submissions, so it is crucial for athletic trainers to keep a record of their continuing education requirements and submission to the BOC for two years after the reporting cycle has closed.

As with all the documents listed earlier, it is imperative that athletic trainers not only keep accurate records but also ensure that they are housed in HIPAA and FERPA compliant databases or storage systems. It is also important that athletic trainers securely retain these documents for at least seven years, though some states have different requirements for retention of records.

Conclusion

Thorough, detailed, and accurate documentation practices are an essential part of athletic training and healthcare at large. Accurate documentation can help ensure clear communication across providers as well as provide the patient with a better understanding of their injury status and recovery timeline. It is no secret that this process can be time-consuming and is one of the least enjoyable aspects of the job as an athletic trainer. However, by adopting sound documentation practices, athletic trainers protect themselves and their institutions against future legal risks while strengthening positive patient outcomes.

CASE STUDY

Allen is a certified athletic trainer at a local high school covering boys' soccer practice. Rick, a high school senior, sustains a knee injury and reports to Allen after practice that he is in severe pain and feels like his left knee is "unstable." Allen conducts a thorough initial evaluation and notes visible swelling and a decrease in range of motion, as well as a positive Lachman's test. Allen suspects an ACL tear after his evaluation but does not communicate that to Rick. Additionally, Allen does not refer Rick to the team physician and opts to treat the injury conservatively with an ice bag. After Rick leaves, Allen quickly documents the injury with the only following information with the intention of returning later to finish documenting Rick's injury:

> Player complains of left knee pain. Swelling observed and ice applied. Rest for three days and return for re-evaluation.

After the three days of rest, Rick returns to practice and forgets to follow up with Allen prior to returning. His knee is still swollen and is still in pain but feels like he can manage the pain. During practice, Rick feels his knee give out again. Instead of returning to the athletic training room, Rick schedules an appointment with an orthopedic doctor. The doctor orders an MRI which shows a complete ACL, grade 2 MCL sprain, and damage to the medial meniscus, and begins discussing the surgical and rehabilitation process with Rick and his parents. Rick and his parents are upset with this news, delayed referral to a physician, and further injury to Rick's knee. As such, they decide to pursue legal action against Allen and the school.

Critical Thinking Questions:

1. What key elements are missing from Allen's documentation that could have provided evidence of appropriate care?
2. What potential legal and ethical consequences might Allen face for his inadequate documentation practices?
3. What documentation strategies should Allen employ to decrease his chances of future legal actions?

References

1. Commission on Accreditation of Athletic Training Education. *Standards and Procedures for Accreditation of Professional Programs in Athletic Training*. 2024. Accessed October 6, 2024. https://caate.net/Portals/0/Standards_and_Procedures_Professional_Programs.pdf?ver=01iHqzdBAW0IsGARUc-19Q%3d%3d
2. Board of Certification for the Athletic Trainer. *Content Outline for Practice Analysis*. 8th ed. Published online March 2023. https://bocatc.org/wp-content/uploads/2024/01/boc-pa8-content-outline-20230109–1.pdf
3. Board of Certification for the Athletic Trainer. *BOC Standards of Professional Practice*. Published online 2023. Accessed October 6, 2024. https://bocatc.org/wp-content/uploads/2024/01/SOPP-2024.pdf

4. Singh H, Naik AD, Rao R, Petersen LA. Reducing Diagnostic Errors through Effective Communication: Harnessing the Power of Information Technology. *Journal of General Internal Medicine*. 2008;23(4):489–494. doi:10.1007/s11606-007-0393-z

5. Rodziewicz TL, Houseman B, Vaqar S, Hipskind JE. Medical Error Reduction and Prevention. In: *StatPearls*. StatPearls Publishing; 2024. Accessed October 15, 2024. http://www.ncbi.nlm.nih.gov/books/NBK499956/

6. Best Practice Guidelines for Athletic Training Documentation. Published online August 2017. https://www.nata.org/sites/default/files/best-practice-guidelines-for-athletic-training-documentation.pdf

7. Sameera V, Bindra A, Rath GP. Human Errors and Their Prevention in Healthcare. *Journal of Anaesthesiology Clinical Pharmacology*. 2021;37(3):328–335. doi:10.4103/joacp.JOACP_364_19

8. Commission on Accreditation of Athletic Training Education. *CAATE Residency and Fellowship Standards*. 2024. Accessed October 6, 2024. https://caate.net/Portals/0/Documents/CAATE-Accreditation-of-Residency-and-Fellowship-Programs.pdf?ver=t8enkWv5FwRikOFXUjbj3Q%3d%3d

9. Podder V, Lew V, Ghassemzadeh S. SOAP Notes. In: *StatPearls*. StatPearls Publishing; 2024. Accessed October 16, 2024. http://www.ncbi.nlm.nih.gov/books/NBK482263/

10. Scarneo-Miller SE, Hosokawa Y, Drezner JA, et al. National Athletic Trainers' Association Position Statement: Emergency Action Plan Development and Implementation in Sport. *Journal of Athletic Training*. 2024;59(6):570-583. doi:10.4085/1062-6050-0521.23

11. BOC Athletic Trainer Life Cycle. *Board of Certification for the Athletic Trainer*. Accessed October 29, 2024. https://bocatc.org/athletic-trainer-life-cycle/

7 Setting-Specific Legal Cases

Chapter Objectives: Following the completion of this chapter, the reader will:

1. List setting-specific common areas of risk.
2. Explain existing case law relevant to athletic training settings.
3. Describe actions that can be taken to mitigate setting-specific risk.

When one thinks of risk management, a number of areas come to mind. For example, identifying conditions that pose the greatest risk for an adverse outcome is essential. These might include but are certainly not limited to, concussions, spinal injuries, fractures, and exertional heat illness. Additionally, risk may be greater in some settings versus others, or at the minimum settings where an athletic trainer works may pose different types of risks. This chapter provides an introduction to some of the more common settings that employ athletic trainers and review examples of case law that pertain to these settings. This is by far not an all-inclusive list, yet it provides an overview that can serve as a starting point for understanding setting-based risk. As you will note, conditions that pose a greater risk may appear in multiple settings.

Secondary School Setting

A strong case can be made that the secondary school setting poses the greatest risk to an athletic trainer. This is a setting where, very often, care and coverage are provided by a single athletic trainer. This individual is responsible for hundreds of student athletes and includes multiple venues of play. Furthermore, each student participating in athletics likely has their own personal family physician, while the employed athletic trainers work under the guidance of their own directing physician. This type of an arrangement exposes one to challenges with proper supervision, timely and thorough informed consent requirements, delayed response times to emergencies, and potential difficulty in carrying out our policies and procedures based on the current standard of care. In this section we highlight a few cases where athletic trainers employed at a secondary school have been named in a claim.

DOI: 10.4324/9781003524823-7

In March of 2017, the First District Appellate Court in Illinois addressed Williams v. Athletico, et al, where the complaint alleged that an athletic trainer failed to assess and evaluate a concussion that was sustained by a male student athlete during a high school football game that took place in 2013.[1] As it is described, the school district hired the company to provide athletic training services, and the company hired the athletic trainer to fulfill the agreement. From a legal perspective, this case establishes the fact that an athletic trainer as a licensed professional who complies with the term "healing art" by way of treating injuries, which has traditionally been referenced to physicians and nurses. This case was filed against a licensed athletic trainer in addition to two organizations that were involved with providing athletic training services to the high school in this case. The claim brought forth by the parents of the now-disabled student athlete alleged the defendants were negligent for failing to perform a proper assessment at the time of the injury on the football field. This assessment related to head trauma and not recognizing a sustained concussion and subsequent inappropriate management of the injury.

Athletic trainers would be wise to learn not only how to work under the standard of care at all times, but also how a court will review their actions. For example, in this case, the court specifically asked the question as to whether or not the standard of care involves procedures that can be conveyed to a lay jury. In doing so, the court also set to determine the extent to which "medical judgment" was necessary as part of the assessment and what type of evidence would be required for the plaintiffs to prove negligence on the part of the athletic trainer. This could include, but may not be limited to, documentation records, one's scope of practice, and even whether or not an expert witness would be necessary. The court essentially ruled that this in fact does fall under the existing "healing art" statue for malpractice as compared to ordinary negligence. This means that the athletic trainer is held to a higher standard. While this type of a case can serve as a precedent to others, it is essential to understand that the language of state licensure differs by state and one has a responsibility of clearly understanding the statute within one's own state of practice. In this case, the court further ruled that the plaintiffs need to establish that the defendants failed to employ the degree of knowledge, skill, and ability that a reasonable athletic trainer would employ under similar circumstances. While this may sound familiar based on readings thus far in this book, all circumstances differ. Nonetheless, the standard-of-care expectations such as proper training, credentialing, planning, and preparation, knowing when to assess, knowing what signs and symptoms to look for with a potential head injury, and knowing how to intervene based upon such findings are all necessary and components that a reasonable athletic trainer should possess. Following the appellate responses, the plaintiffs reserved the right to refile their claim.

As an athletic trainer, would you do anything specific within your practice if you were in a similar setting? How has learning about this lawsuit made you think differently or has it not at all?

Let's take a look at another secondary school setting lawsuit that occurred in the State of Oregon. In 2018, the parents of a 17-year-old Oregon high school football player sued the Hermiston School District for $38 million dollars following a concussion injury.[2]

In this suit, the plaintiffs claimed that the defendants failed to properly respond to a concussion that their son had sustained and as a result now has permanent brain damage. As you should recall, finding damage and establishing a relationship between one's actions and the damage are essential components of negligence. The plaintiffs further allege that nobody at the high school treated their son for a concussion or informed them as parents that such was the injury following a helmet-to-helmet collision from a year previous in a junior varsity football game at the age of 15. The suit further alleges that the district's athletic trainer cleared their son to play four days after the initial hit to the head despite claims of lingering concussion-like symptoms. It was reported that in a subsequent game he encountered repeated contact to his head that ultimately rendered him unconscious. The teen's mother stated that just a few hours later at home she noticed him curled up in a fetal position on his couch crying from a severe headache and that he was unable to walk steadily without falling. He also vomited throughout the same night.

With respect to permanent damages, the parents claim that their son still suffers from vision disturbances, headaches, and especially balance difficulties that have led to numerous falls and more injuries preventing him from attending school on a full-time basis. He is unable to drive a car or take part in previously enjoyed hobbies such as bowling or hunting.

Of particular note in this case is the state in which the claim is filed. In 2009, "Max's Law" was signed into legislation, named after Max Conradt, a 17-year-old high school quarterback who suffered a concussion and was cleared to play soon after in a future game. He subsequently collapsed at half-time later diagnosed with internal cranial bleeding, lapsed into a coma for a period of three months, and emerged with permanent brain damage. Max's Law specifically prohibits players from being cleared to return to a game following suspicion of a concussion without a medical professional thoroughly examining the situation and providing such clearance. The law also mandates training for all coaches regarding the recognition of signs and symptoms of a concussion. As you can see, similar precedent was set in the very same state. In this case, the parents state that their son was removed from the football game because the coach felt he was disoriented and couldn't remember the plays. These are obvious symptoms of a sport-related concussion that every athletic trainer should recognize. The claim also notes that the teen returned to play in a following game despite not being seen and cleared by a medical professional.

In this lawsuit, like most others of similar circumstances, the plaintiff sought damages that included payment for past and future medical expenses, daily professional personal assistance, lost wages associated with future employment and earning capabilities, and psychiatric care for anxiety and depression. The case was ultimately settled for $38.9 million.

As an athletic trainer, what steps would you have taken to avoid finding yourself in situation like this? Take a moment to ask yourself and jot down your response. After you do so, continue to read on.

An obvious thought would be to perform a thorough concussion assessment with follow-up care and a required physician evaluation prior to initiating a graded return-to-play process. A better strategy would be to establish a complete concussion management program, thereby using policies and procedures the help you in risk management. This includes, but is not limited to, policies that align with the most current position statements and existing legislation, documented education provided to all stakeholders, adherence to procedures laid out in the policy, appropriate physician assessment and clearance when ready, and a closely monitored graded return to play with informed consent along the way.

Now let's look at one more case that involves a secondary school athlete, this one in San Marcos, California. This case also involves a concussion. While this is certainly commonplace, not all lawsuits in this setting do involve concussions as we have seen cases filed from exertional heat illness deaths, deaths from lightning strikes, and others.

In the Eveland vs. City of San Marcos case, Scott Eveland was a senior linebacker for Mission Hills High School not far from San Diego.[3] Mission Hills School is overseen by the San Marcos Unified School District. Of interest in this particular case are statements made by some of those involved in the incident itself that led to the injury. Some 250 depositions were reported to be taken of various witnesses. One former athletic training student claimed that the football team's head coach ignored signs of distress that the teen player displayed. She also stated that for a week prior to the actual incident he complained to the team's athletic trainer about having headaches. These headaches in fact held him out of some practice activities, Minutes before the actual game began where he apparently sustained his head injury, he asked whether he could sit out of the first quarter since his head was hurting. He states that the coach refused to take him out.

In the end, and approximately four years later, both sides reached a settlement in the amount of $5 million to support the victim for the remainder of his life under disabled living circumstances as he communicates through the use of an iPad/keyboard and mobilizes via a wheelchair. The San Marcos Unified School District also did not admit to any responsibility in the settlement. In fact, a joint statement by both parties following the announcement of the settlement read as such:

> *Scott Eveland and his family agree that this settlement does not suggest that the professional and hard-working coaches, athletic trainers, administrators, and staff at Mission Hills High School intentionally contributed to the unfortunate and tragic accident that occurred during a high school football game.*

In this case, the importance of communication and documentation is essential. Furthermore, as noted in previous cases discussed, the act of following the appropriate standard of care cannot be underemphasized. Accidents will happen. Injuries will happen. Some of these will not have a positive outcome. When they don't have a positive outcome, there is a strong likelihood that a lawsuit will be filed. If so, your best form of defense is a strong case of offense whereby you were prepared and did your job within your scope and to the highest ethical and legal standards using best practices.

It should be clear that despite each of these aforementioned cases taking place in a high school setting, these occurrences can realistically happen in any other setting for that matter. As always, issues of standard of care, omission, commission, informed consent, duty, etc., are all hallmark necessities for every athletic trainer, regardless of practice setting.

Intercollegiate Setting

In the case of Augustus Feleccia and Justin T. Resch versus Lackawanna College in 2018 we explore a case of gross negligence. Unfortunately, this pattern of events may not be all that rare, especially when proper credentialing and licensing of athletic trainers are ignored.[4]

This incident took place in Pennsylvania and was argued in court many years later. Two student athletes who played Football at Lackawanna Junior College (LJC) claimed gross negligence and recklessness on behalf of the school for allowing unlicensed personnel to perform the duties when not proven to be qualified. As mentioned, this case sounds all too unfamiliar to athletic trainers. At LJC the athletic director (AD) typically hired two athletic trainers to provide care and coverage for the football team. One particular year the AD hired two recently graduated athletic trainers who had not yet passed their certification examination and thus therefore were also not yet licensed in the state as is required of all athletic trainers in Pennsylvania. At the start of their official employment at LJC, both received notice that they had not passed their certification exams. As a result, the AD retitled their job descriptions previously agreed upon from "athletic trainer" to "first responder." However, neither of the two new employees executed revised job descriptions. At the start of football practice and at the time when contact drills were performed, the student athletes were aware of the athletic trainers not passing their certification exams. While participating in the classic "Oklahoma Drill" where individuals go full contact head-to-head, both of the named student athletes were injured. One of the student athletes sustained a T-7 vertebral fracture and the other an acute brachial plexus injury, oftentimes referred to as a "stinger." One of the athletic trainers cleared the student athlete with the stinger to practice once he noted that he "felt better." Certainly, one of the items that came into question was whether or not the individuals were qualified to work in the role of a licensed and certified athletic trainer. Where this came into play in the courts related to an injury liability waiver that the school provided informing the student athletes that they were at inherent risk of an injury while playing football. The courts also looked into the question of the responsibility of the school to provide proper care and administer safety measures to assure an environment that minimizes risk. As part of doing so, the school acknowledged in its policies that it provides certified athletic trainers in this particular role which coincides with the practice of a licensed and certified athletic trainer in the Commonwealth of Pennsylvania. The appellate court did in fact rule that LJC had a duty to provide licensed and certified athletic trainers for student athletes participating in their athletic programs and such duty was breached. Do the words "duty" and "breached" ring a bell? They should, as they are two of the four requirements for negligence to be found. The appellate court found negligence, but not necessarily "gross negligence" or "recklessness," which they stated is held to a higher bar in such that proof is needed to demonstrate that the act or non-act was intentional and designed to harm others.

At this point you are probably asking yourself "why was this case so complicated?" "How could they even be allowed to hire an athletic trainer who didn't pass one's exam and is not licensed?" In an ideal world, where common sense rules, you are correct. Have you ever heard of a classmate or colleague being hired pending their certification results? The pressure on this person is immense. What happened if they did not pass? Were they no longer hired? Were they hired under a different role as in this case? Did they carry out the revised role or did they still act as if they were certified and licensed and left others with the same perception of such? Ask yourself this question—in this case, if the athletic trainers (who by completion of their degree they earned that title) were not certified nor licensed, revised and signed a different role and function until they were appropriately credentialed, informed all stakeholders, and acted as such in the role of a first responder, would there be any negligence in this case if all they did was respond to the injuries and triage to healthcare providers? Everything is not always so clear, and even when one believes to be acting appropriately and in the best interest of others, things can go wrong, be interpreted differently, and find one defending their actions. What would you do in a case like this where you signed on to a new job but you didn't pass your examination. Would you still be anxious to work? Perhaps you were especially tempted to work in any role because of the long-awaited anticipation as well as the much-needed paycheck? What if you were the employer? What would you do if you were the AD and this occurred? Would you revise one's role from athletic trainer to first responder and be comfortable with that? How would you explain this to coaches, players, maybe even messaging to parents? Do you think that raises any levels of concern amongst any of them? What about if you were one of the players? How would you feel? Do you think this happens in medicine when a doctor does not pass the medical boards? What about for paramedics or emergency medical technicians? These are all questions you should consider in any job you take as an athletic trainer. Regardless, once you are certified and licensed you should always make decisions with ethical and legal considerations in mind and how they impact all potential stakeholders.

Now let's look at some cases that took place in a college/University setting but again could truthfully happen in any athletic training setting. The next two cases that we will discuss involve inappropriate behavior alleged on the part of the athletic trainer employed by the college athletics department.

The first case we will discuss involves alleged misconduct by an athletic trainer at North Carolina State University. We will highlight this case as it represents a different type of claim and also demonstrates a different outcome and the attention drawn to it from the media.[5]

A number of student athletes came forward to the state and eventually filed federal claims that one of the staff athletic trainers inappropriately touched them during treatment sessions over the period of a couple of years and therefore sexually

abused them. It was noted in the claim that they felt the athletic trainer was groom-
ing certain athletes during massage treatments. Based on the alleged misconduct,
lawyers for the plaintiffs claimed this created a hostile working environment.
The lawsuits specifically stated that the athletic trainer performed massages and
touched the student athletes' genitals on multiple occasions without medical need
or the student's consent. One of the lawsuits states that this occurred as many as
100 times. The lawsuits claim that the University was aware of the athletic trainer's behavior and failed to comply with federal Title IX regulations and its own
non-discrimination policy. When the suit was filed, internal investigations were
performed and the athletic trainer was placed on administrative leave. Numerous
media outlets in print, online, and on television carried this story and reported on
the filed lawsuits. The plaintiffs came out on television interviews and said their
goal was to not let this happen to future student athletes. Plaintiff's lawyers spoke
out and claimed the alleged abuse was systemic. The defense argued that with such
allegations the complainants did not refuse to continue to work with the athletic
trainer.

Initially one of the lawsuits also sued the University, its Chancellor, director of
athletics, and senior associate athletic director. These individuals were later dismissed as defendants by one of the judges. Despite witnesses stating that they
informed the administration of their concerns, the judge in the case ruled that the
allegations were absent of a "specific incident" and therefore dismissed the claims
in favor of the University. The University also argued that it had no knowledge of
the alleged behavior until the lawsuit was filed and did not ignore any suggested
complaints by coaches, athletes, or others.

There are a number of learning points within the framework of this case for
athletic trainers to consider. To begin with, understand that with any allegation
of wrongdoing, and perhaps especially of the sexual misconduct nature, head-
lines will be drawn and potentially dominate the news cycle for a period of time.
Regardless whether one is innocent or guilty of such charges, the news coverage
will still be presented as if they certainly may have been despite careful language
of the term "alleged." Some say that there is no such thing as bad press, in that any
press is good press. This might be a situation where such is not the case. This is of
utmost interest because if you were to perform an internet search about this case,
you will in fact find a plethora of links about the alleged incident. However, you
will not find the same volume of stories that speak to the outcome and dismissal.
Regardless of a legal dismissal, and whether or not the acts did or did not occur,
the named athletic trainer will face a difficult time moving forward career-wise as a
result of the extensive negatively directed media. If this were you, how would you
proceed in a job search and explain such circumstances?

Another thing to consider is the timeline between the alleged accusations of
wrongdoing and when the lawsuit was filed. This is not uncommon. While with
blatantly negligent situations claims can be brought forth rather expediently, oftentimes years can go by before a legal suit is filed. This emphasizes the importance
of thorough documentation as it is not likely one can remember details of activities

that may have occurred some two years ago. In addition, one may still be employed and working, thus requiring an individual to remain focused enough to continue to provide competent care for their patients or athletes. Or, the individual may be placed on administrative leave—with or without pay—pending the outcome of the investigation and litigation. Again, if this were you, what would you do during the time while you were on administrative leave not knowing how long that could last?

Once again, ask yourself how you would react if you were accused of an inappropriate sexual behavior with an athlete from treatments you performed years ago. Remembering back to earlier readings in this book, who would you contact first? How many people and who specifically would you tell? How do you think your life would change? If you were on paid administrative leave for any extended period of time, what would you do during this time? If you were found not to be negligent of the charges, do you think you would have any difficulties returning to work or seeking a new position elsewhere?

The next case to review also took place in a collegiate athletic setting. In this case, filed in 2023, a male athletic trainer was accused of committing sexual assaults toward female student athletes over a period of several years.[6-9] At least four female student athletes made the claims and stated the athletic trainer also groomed multiple players during the same timeframe. The plaintiffs stated that the alleged acts occurred in the athletic training room, offices, on buses, and in the defendant's private hotel rooms during away trips to games. These claimants further documented that instead of providing what they thought would be 10-minute sports massages, the athletic trainer performed full-body massages in a private room that could last for hours in length. They also stated that they were threatened by the athletic trainer if they ever "said anything bad about him" in that if he "goes down they would all go down with him."

When the alleged misconduct was first reported, the University notified law enforcement and removed the athletic trainer from his job duties pending a thorough five-month investigation. The findings subsequently reported that the athletic trainer was found responsible for violating University policies and he was therefore terminated from his position. The final report also found that the department had no written policies or procedures regarding proper athletic trainer conduct, setting boundaries with athletes, or working with athletes of the opposite sex. In the lawsuits, the women are seeking financial compensation for damages related to psychological pain and suffering, medical bills, counseling, other miscellaneous costs, and punitive damages.

The supervisor of the athletic trainer defendant, also an athletic trainer, was accused of negligence for his failure to investigate the situation, provide adequate training to the coaches, implement safety measures, or safeguard the women from the alleged abuse. Similarly, the University was alleged to have failed to supervise the staff athletic trainer effectively and therefore ensure student athletes' safety. It was further alleged that the University was aware of the athletic trainer's conduct but failed to take any necessary action. Of interest is that the lawsuit claimed that the University tipped off the athletic trainer about the ongoing investigation prior to notifying law enforcement. The athletic trainer possessed a university-administered cell phone that allegedly stored potentially incriminating photographs and videos. The lawsuit was filed for "in excess of $75,000 " in damages and also sought the following actions be implemented:

- The University establish safety protocols
- The University contact former student athletes to identify any additional alleged victims
- Prevent the athletic trainer from retaining his state licensure

As of the preparation of this chapter manuscript in 2024, a federal judge has denied the University's motion to dismiss the lawsuit.[10] Of interest in the judge's ruling is that the case would not be considered "medical malpractice" in that sexual abuse is not medical care and is not related to whether or not the provider gave adequate care. The judge cited *Fairbanks Hosp. v. Harrold,* 895 N.E.2d 732 (Ind. Ct. App. 2008 in the ruling.[11] The judge also stated that negligent supervision of a sexual abuser is also not medical malpractice and cited *Indiana Dep't of Ins. v. Doe*, 211 N.E.3d 1014 (Ind. Ct. App. 2023).[12]

The next collegiate setting case describes a former baseball player who filed a malpractice lawsuit alleging negligence against a University sports medicine staff claiming the treatment received following a lower leg injury in 2016 fell below the accepted standard of care for a reasonably prudent athletic program. The lawsuit asserts the alleged improper actions and inactions cost the student athlete his baseball career and led to sustained physical ailments and inconveniences.[13]

Orthopedic physician examination reported that the student athlete had an accessory soleus muscle, something seen as rare as 6% of the overall population.[14] In 2016, the accessory muscle was excised surgically. The lawsuit outlined that treatment for the injury included dry-needling, thermal therapy, and restricted activity while performing baseball fielding drills in a protective ankle boot. The lawsuit claims that the treatment interventions contradicted the recommendations of the surgeon. The plaintiff asserted that for four months following the surgery he was not seen by a physician and that his lack of progress was attributed to being psychological on his part. During an eventual postoperative visit with the physician, tests revealed potential nerve damage and significant deficits. The physician recommended intensive rehabilitation to address the concerns and an independent consultation with a different rehabilitation provider. The student athlete's scholarship was later revoked. Continued care was provided by an external private practice and he subsequently had surgery on both his hip and ankle which may or may not be related to the original injury recovery process.

The lawsuit in this case seeks damages for loss of past, present, and future enjoyment of life, past, present, and future medical expenses, loss of income earnings and opportunities, mental anguish, pain and suffering, and loss of mobility. At the time of this writing, the case has not been publicly reported to be resolved. As an athletic trainer, you can probably identify with numerous postoperative cases that do not proceed as planned. This will happen, unfortunately, as not all outcomes will be favorable. From a risk management perspective, the key is for you to be able to ensure you have done everything you could have according to the standard of care and as such documented all aspects of the case. Can you recall a situation where a student athlete in a college athletics setting underwent a surgery and did not recover according to plan? How involved were you in the rehabilitation process? Did you communicate in a timely and effective manner with all parties—physicians, coaches, parents, student athlete? Would you have done anything differently? Was your documentation thorough? Would it be able to show progress or regress in an objective manner with data? Did you respond to the student athlete's feedback? These are the types of things every athletic trainer should consider with every case regardless of setting or type of injury.

For the next case, let's stay in the collegiate setting but now focus on a cheerleading injury that occurred at Southeastern University in Florida.[15] A former cheerlead sued the school, the former coach, and the assistant athletic trainer for negligence following multiple concussions where she alleged she did not receive adequate care. The lawsuit specifically claims that the University did not properly train stakeholders on concussion protocols in place in accordance with the governing body the National Association of Intercollegiate Athletics (NAIA).

The cheerleader apparently fell on her head during a team practice in 2016 while performing an acrobatic maneuver. The assistant coach of the cheerleading squad was the first to attend to the cheerleader. Deposition testimony stated that she did not show any signs or symptoms of a concussion and after practice she was driven home by the coach without seeing an athletic trainer or physician. A subsequent fall approximately a month later led to ongoing neurocognitive deficits according to the claim. It was asserted that the cheerleader suffered a total of four concussions to date and that the University policy states that after a third concussion a referral to a physician is required for further assessment prior to any clearance to return to participation.

Of interest in this case is the claim that just a year prior to this incident, nine cheerleaders requested a meeting with the University administration to voice concerns over their perceived lack of concern for the team's safety by the coach, in that they were forced to perform certain stunts and tumbles despite having existing injuries. The lawyers for the plaintiff further noted several other cases of student athletes not being treated appropriately with concussion-related signs and symptoms. These claims noted that the individuals were either forced or encouraged to return to play without a proper physician evaluation for safe clearance. The lawyers additionally referred to text messages from the school's athletic trainers identifying cases where players were not properly screened or were allowed to continue to play despite having concussion-related symptoms.

If you were the athletic trainer in this case, and you learned of being named in a lawsuit for alleged inappropriate concussion protocol actions and inactions, what would be your first response? What exactly would go through your mind? Who would you contact in what order? Exactly how much information and what details would you share? Would you go back and look at the medical records of the plaintiffs to see if you can recall each incident?

Professional Sports Setting

For the next case we will turn to the National Football League (NFL) where in 2013 a former kicker sued his team for $20 million claiming that his career ended due to acquiring an infection (MRSA—methicillin-resistant staphylococcus aureus) in the big toe of his kicking foot and stated that the athletic trainer was the source of the infection.[16–18]

The kicker had the nail of his big toe trimmed by the athletic trainer as he does annually, and he noted on this particular occasion that two days later he ran a fever while the toe appeared red and swollen. An infection ensued and the kicker attributed this to "unsanitary conditions" of the facility while failing to employ necessary sterile techniques and routinely leaving therapy devices, equipment, and surfaces unclean. The lawsuit also claims that the kicker may have acquired the infection from the athletic trainer himself who apparently previously had his own case of MRSA. The lawsuit also alleges that previous incidences of infections occurred to players but that the team "failed to disclose such incidences." The case sought financial damages to include future lost earnings.

The kicker said he became concerned after a number of days without improvement and sought an outside physician for another opinion. The kicker subsequently underwent three surgeries to his toe and had a central line inserted for six weeks of antibiotic treatment.

The case was ultimately settled approximately two years after the lawsuit was filed with the final terms of the settlement undisclosed.

Have you ever seen or treated an athlete or patient with MRSA? If so, do you know how the infection was acquired? Do you think the facility or lack of cleanliness and sterile techniques could have led to the infection? What about the current settings you are immersed in clinically? How aware are you of policies and procedures to maintain a sterile healthcare facility? Are you familiar with the standards for maintaining a clean facility?[19]

Rehabilitation Clinical Setting

The next case we will discuss took place in a physical therapy clinic. The clinic employed physical therapists, physical therapist assistants, and athletic trainers. A high school student claimed improper management during treatment and failure to supervise the rehabilitation interventions that led to a reinjury and subsequent loss of a college scholarship.[20]

The high school basketball player was undergoing rehabilitation in the private clinic following surgery for an anterior cruciate ligament tear. His surgeon prescribed physical therapy 2–3 times a week for a total of 12 weeks. The male athlete discontinued going to therapy on his own accord after eight weeks unbeknown to his parents. Following the month's absence, he returned with significant deficits in his functional status. He participated in six more weeks of therapy and was then discharged. At the completion of his final visit, he was cleared by his orthopedic surgeon to return to sports without restrictions. At this time, the patient opted to continue exercise activity at a local gym 4–5 days/week and subsequently decreased the number of gym visits over the next few months. He reported consistent mild pain and occasional throbbing near the end of each day though not reported to the healthcare providers.

The next visit that the athlete had with a healthcare provider took place approximately two months prior to the upcoming basketball season. The goal was to seek guidance on continued training to optimize preparedness for the upcoming season. This took place approximately three months after the last formal visit, and at this time, the patient did not report any concerns with the knee. During this visit, the physical therapist assistant had the patient perform a box jump landing on one foot, which the patient said he had not done before, and upon completing the third one "felt his knee collapse." Clinical staff testified in fact that the patient did perform this test months ago as part of the criteria for discharge and return to full activity.

Further examination revealed a bucket handle-type tear to the patient's meniscus that led to two additional surgeries. These surgeries and the postoperative rehabilitation prevented the individual from playing his senior season of high school basketball. Hence, the lawsuit that was filed naming the clinic and the PTA specifically claimed (1) a failure to properly assess and evaluate, (2) a failure to prescribe and implement a proper treatment plan and protocol, and (3) a failure to properly supervise the PTA that led to reinjury. The loss claimed in the suit by the plaintiff was that he had multiple Division 1 scholarship offers prior to the reinjury that were no longer offered to him and that any school that reached out for him to play at the college level did not offer any scholarship money. The plaintiff claimed that the opportunity to chase his dreams of playing basketball at the next level was lost and sought over $300,000 due to his parents' loss of income, medical bills, and cost of tuition, room, and board.

This case brings up a number of interesting items to discuss. For context, one can easily imagine an athletic trainer in the same role as the PTA and performing somewhat similar responsibilities of patient care in a rehabilitation clinic. The plaintiffs stated that they chose the private practice due to the advertising claims of expertise by the physical therapist, but instead were not assessed nor treated by such a person, and instead managed by other personnel with less than the same promoted level of expertise. Again, one can relate this case very easily to an athletic trainer employed in a similar setting.

In this case, documentation supported the defendant's claim on what was performed and how the reinjury may have occurred, with witnesses in support of the defendant's testimony. This is important as the only version of the injury being reported as it was by the plaintiff was from the plaintiff himself. With that said, there was a question as to whether or not adequate musculoskeletal screening was performed prior to administering the testing as a significant amount of time had lapsed since the last complete formal evaluation.

Of interest in this case is that despite filing the lawsuit, the plaintiff went on to play basketball at a Division 2 for two years and then transferred to a Division 1 college. Thus, as you recall one of the requirements for negligence is damage. It could be argued that no damage was established on behalf of the defendants in this case and that it is not uncommon at all for one to have a knee surgery and not return to the same level of play. This athlete did in fact return to play and thus the burden to establish negligence or malpractice would become much more difficult.

In addition, the plaintiff ultimately dropped the clinicians from the lawsuit, but did not dismiss the claim regarding the alleged "false advertising." Nonetheless a settlement was ultimately reached for a much smaller amount.

This case highlights a couple of areas for athletic trainers to consider when working in a private practice clinical setting that also translates to all other settings. To begin with, thorough documentation is always helpful, including informed consent especially with a minor, and details of both objective and subjective findings and activities. This also includes documentation when a patient is non-compliant or absent for expected treatment sessions. Proper supervision is always necessary according to the standard of care and one's practice act. It is a good practice to assure that when you introduce yourself you also make it clear to the patient what your practicing credentials are in a way that is not misleading. While representing oneself appropriately is good practice, it is rare that a lawsuit is generated as is in this case where the marketing use of a word or term is not equally perceived by the patient as receiving that same level of care. For example, you may find private practice clinics with the words "elite," or something similar in their title. It is not common that a patient will therefore define the term "elite" in their own mind and then equate that to a certain level of care. In this case, what they were really saying is that the clinic used the terms to essentially promote the owner and that person's skills and experience and instead were treated by other staff with less experience.

Summary

In highlighting a few cases that involved an athletic trainer and alleged negligence based on different settings, one should be able to recognize how such claims can occur essentially in any setting and that the common theme for all risk management is to have thorough policies and procedures, adhere to all professional standards of care and practice act guidelines, and implement complete documentation approaches and communication skills among other areas of consideration.

References

1. *Williams v. Athletico*, LTD. Justia US Law 2017 IL App (1st) 161902. Accessed February 16, 2024.   https://law.justia.com/cases/illinois/court-of-appeals-first-appellate-district/201 7/1-16-1902.html.
2. Oregon High School Football Player Sues for $38 Million after Suffering Concussion. *The Oregonian*. September 13, 2018. Accessed March 20, 2024. https://www.oregon-live.com/pacific-northwest-news/2018/09/38_million_lawsuit_football_pl.html.
3. Eveland Settles Head Injury Case for $4.375 Million. *The San Diego Union-Tribune*. March 9, 2012. Accessed February 19, 2024. https://www.sandiegouniontribune.com/ sdut-eveland-settles-head-injury-case-4375-million-2012mar09-htmlstory.html.
4. *Feleccia v. Lackawanna College, et al.*, Justia US Law Supreme Court of Pennsylvania Middle District (J-96–2018). August 20, 2019. Accessed March 20, 2024. https://law. justia.com/cases/pennsylvania/supreme-court/2019/75-map–2017.html.

5. Another Former Athlete Sues N.C. State Alleging Athletic Trainer Misconduct. *Paul Steibach Athletic Business.* February 3, 2023. Accessed March 2, 2024. https://www.athleticbusiness.com/operations/legal/article/15306416/another-former-athlete-sues-nc-state-alleging-athletic-trainer-misconduct.

6. Former Butler Athletic Trainer Accused of Abusing Female Athletes in Federal Lawsuit. *WFYI News Indianapolis.* July 27, 2023. Accessed March 26, 2024. https://www.wfyi.org/news/articles/3-butler-university-soccer-players-federal-lawsuit-alleging-abuse.

7. https://www.lawow.org/doe-v-butler-university-et-al-2023-07-26

8. Fourth Women's Soccer Player Sues Butler for Alleged Sexual Assault by Athletic Trainer. *The Athletic Katie Strang.* August 18, 2023. Accessed March 27, 2024. https://theathletic.com/4787904/2023/08/18/butler-womens-soccer-lawsuit/.

9. Butler Athlete Says Trainer's Sexual Assaults Were "Frequent", over a "Long Period of Time". *Indy StarAkeem Glaspie.* July 26, 2023. Accessed March 19, 2024. https://www.indystar.com/story/sports/college/butler/2023/07/26/former-butler-athletic-trainer-accused-of-abusing-3-female-athletes/70471395007/.

10. Federal Judge Denies Butler's Motion to Dismiss Student-athletes' Sexual Abuse Case against Former Athletic Trainer. *The Indiana Lawyer Danial Carson.* January 23, 2024. Accessed March 27, 2024. https://www.theindianalawyer.com/articles/federal-judge-denies-butlers-motion-to-dismiss-student-athletes-sexual-abuse-case-against-former-athletic-trainer.

11. *Fairbanks v. Harrold*, 895 N.E. 2d 732. Accessed March 27, 2024. https://casetext.com/case/fairbanks-v-harrold.

12. *Doe v. Butler University*, 1:23-CV-01302-JRS-MKK. Accessed March 27, 2024. *Indiana Dep't of Ins. v. Doe*, 211 N.E.3d 1014 (Ind. Ct. App. 2023).

13. Former Clemson Baseball Player Grant Fox Files Malpractice Lawsuit against University. *Manie Robinson Greenville News.* February 24, 2024. Accessed March 27, 2024. https://www.greenvilleonline.com/story/sports/college/clemson/2019/02/22/clemson-former-player-medical-malpractice-lawsuit/2948974002/.

14. Reddy P, Mccollum GA. The Accessory Soleus Muscle Causing Tibial Nerve Compression Neuropathy: A Case Report. *The South African Orthopaedic Journal.* 2015; 14(4):58–61.

15. Former Cheerleader Ali Roberts Sues Southeastern University in Lakeland for Negligence, Says She Didn't Receive Proper Care after Suffering Concussions. *Ray Beasock the Ledger.* March 5, 2019. Accessed March 27, 2024. https://www.theledger.com/story/news/2019/03/05/cheerleader-roberts-southeastern-university-lakeland-negligence-receive-proper-suffering-concussions/53187834007/.

16. Former NFL Player's Suit Blames Athletic Trainer for MRSA. *Training & Conditioning.* April 9, 2015. Accessed March 27, 2024. https://training-conditioning.com/news/former-nfl-player-s-suit-blames-athletic-trainer-for-mrsa/.

17. Lawrence Tynes Says MRSA Infection Ended NFL Career. *Pat Yasinskas ESPN.* April 6, 2015. Accessed March 27, 2024. https://www.espn.com/nfl/story/_/id/12632029/lawrence-tynes-sues-tampa-bay-buccaneers-claiming-mrsa-infection-ended-career.

18. Bucaneers, Lawrence Tynes Reach Settlement in MRSA Lawsuit. *Alec Nathan Bleacher Report.* February 21, 2017. Accessed March 27, 2024. https://bleacherreport.com/articles/2694322-buccaneers-lawrence-tynes-reach-settlement-in-mrsa-lawsuit.

19. *BOC Facility Principles Document & Online Resources.* Accessed March 27, 2024. https://bocatc.org/public-protection/standards-discipline/standards-discipline/facility-principles.

20. Physical Therapist Case Study: High School Athlete Alleges Loss of College Scholarship Due to Reinjury during Treatment. *Presented by HPSO and CBA.* Accessed March 27, 2024. https://www.hpso.com/Resources/Legal-and-Ethical-Issues/Athlete-alleges-loss-of-scholarship-due-to-reinjury-during-physical-therapy

8   Clinical Topic-Specific Cases

Chapter Objectives: Following the completion of this chapter, the reader will:

1. Understand legal issues associated with specific injuries or areas of practice.
2. Recognize case law associated with specific injuries or areas of practice.
3. Understand how to develop risk management policies and procedures based on specific case law associated with specific injuries or areas of practice.

Introduction

This chapter presents case law that is directly related to either specific injuries or potential problem areas associated with those injuries. The topics covered include concussion, exertional heat illness, and drug testing that are heavily influenced by written law. Cases related to falls or burns in therapy settings are also covered. The intent of the chapter is to give a broad overview, supported by case law, of each of the specific areas as opposed to an in-depth discussion of the topics.

Concussion

In 2006, Zackery Lystedt was 13-year-old middle school student and played football at Tahoma Junior High School in Washington.[1] During the second quarter of the game, Zackery hit his head on the ground after tackling an opponent. He came out of the game and remained on the bench until the second half. Zackery later returned to play in the third quarter and completed the game. Shortly after the game, Zackery collapsed and was taken to a hospital. After the injury, Zackery remained in a coma for 31 days, was unable to speak for 9 months, and had to be fed through a tube for almost two years.

The injury suffered by Zackery Lystedt was the driving force behind the implementation of a law in Washington requiring athletes that suffer head injuries to be evaluated by a medical professional before being allowed to return to play. Currently, all 50 states[2] have enacted laws dictating that student athletes must be evaluated by medical personnel before returning to play. The family of Zackery Lystedt reached a settlement with Tahoma Schools but Zackery will live with physical challenges due to the injury for the rest of his life.[1]

DOI: 10.4324/9781003524823-8

Adrian Arrington was a college football player at Eastern Illinois University. Arrington suffered multiple concussion episodes during his college career and returned to play after each of them. Eventually, Adrian developed symptoms associated with brain injury including seizures and blackouts. Adrian brought suit against the NCAA for failure to provide adequate care of him after suffering each concussion. Arrington and the NCAA eventually reached a settlement that resulted in requiring baseline testing and not allowing a player with a concussion to return to play on that same day[3]

When Mike Webster died, he was virtually homeless, living in his vehicle or, very often, under an overpass. He had the appearance of a homeless person with mental health issues. "Iron Mike" Webster played 220 games for the Pittsburgh Steelers and was one of the tough guys. He also suffered from the effects of multiple concussions over his career.[4] So much so, that his quality of life plummeted during his last years.

Mike Webster's story was one of the key factors that initiated the move toward a settlement between the National Football League and former players. The NFL and former players reached an agreement[5] to compensate players for damages they sustained from concussions. As of the writing of this text, 1,624 claims have been paid by the NFL for a total of just over 1.3 million dollars.[6]

Exertional Heat Illness

According to the Annual Football Fatality Survey[7] over 70 football athletes have died due to exertional heat illness since 1996. When broken down by setting or level of play, 52 were at the high school level, 15 occurred in college players, while two professional players died and three middle school or rec sport players died. Death due to exertional heat illness is very preventable and a proactive approach to prevention is recommended by an interprofessional group of experts.[8] Unfortunately, however, there are examples of case law centering on exertional heat illness.

One of the higher profile exertional heat illness cases involved Korey Stringer, who played offensive tackle for the Minnesota Vikings.[9] Stringer began to have problems on the first day of practice when he reported to the medical staff that he had an upset stomach. Later during practice that day, Stringer vomited but continued to practice. The heat index that day was estimated to be 109. Stringer experienced difficulty in practice the following morning, in a practice in which the heat index was estimated to be over 90. The practice ended at 11:15 and Stringer's condition began to slowly deteriorate. He was taken to the trailer that served as an on-field athletic training room. At 12:08 PM Stringer was transported, by ambulance, to a hospital. The ambulance arrived at the hospital at 12:24 PM. At 12:35, Stringer's temperature reading was 108.8. At 1:20 PM Stringer, now in cardiac arrest, was administered CPR. At 1:50 PM on August 1, 2001, Korey Stringer was pronounced dead by the medical staff in the hospital.

Kelci Stringer, the wife of the deceased player, brought a wrongful death suit against the Minnesota Vikings and members of the medical staff, individually. This case is a tragic reminder exertional heat illness can impact athletes at any level of competition. While the case itself represents a tragic loss to the Stringer family it also served as the genesis for developing the Korey String Institute.[10] The Korey Stringer Institute was established by the University of Connecticut, in conjunction with Stringer's widow, Kelci, and the National Football League. Since its inception, the Stringer Institute has become a driving force in research and education on exertional heat illness.

In July of 2017, Patrick Clancy was participating in a pre-season soccer practice at Monticello High School, in Charlottesville, Virginia. During practice that day the heat index was estimated to be in the range of what the National Weather Service identifies as extreme danger.[11] When Clancy eventually returned home after practice his parents tried to cool him down. When those efforts failed, and Clancy's condition began to worsen, they took him to a local emergency clinic where he was treated for exertional heat illness. The episode left Clancy with some level of permanent damage and the family initiated a suit against the school and coaches.

Failure to follow established guidelines very likely played a role in the death of Travis Stowers, a high school student in Indiana.[12] Guidelines published by the Indiana State High School Activities Association state that pre-season practices can only be 180 minutes in length. The association also has guidelines for allowable rest times between two-a-day practices. Both of these policies were violated during the events that led to Stowers' death. After a lengthy legal battle in which the initial court ruling was in favor of the school, the case was ultimately reversed, to the benefit of the Stowers family.[13]

In one of the more high-profile [14] cases, Justin McNair experienced an exertional heat illness episode on May 29, 2018, that ultimately resulted in his death. The University of Maryland employed Rod Walters of Walters, Inc., consulting to evaluate and report on the episode. The hiring of a consultant is a significant factor in that it creates an external document that provides much more information than is typically found in a standard legal case. The published timeline from that day indicates that Justin began to demonstrate heat-related symptoms at 4:53 PM and was eventually transported to the hospital at 6:36 pm that day.

The Walters report is extensive and provides an in-depth look at everything that transpired during the event. The report goes further in that it not only addresses shortcomings of individuals and the system that was in place but also speaks to the very nature of the existing athletic healthcare delivery system as well. The document points out that, like many other athletic healthcare delivery systems, coaches maintain a supervisory role over athletic trainers. As mentioned in the risk management chapter, the ideal system is one in which athletic trainers report directly to a physician or other healthcare provider and not a coach or athletic director.

Burns

Providing care to a patient or athlete is accompanied by a responsibility to do no harm. One example of an adverse reaction associated with direct patient care is that of a burn to one's skin. It is safe to see that burns are not the result of intentional acts, but rather unintentional acts of commission or omission. Interventions with therapeutic modalities such as heat packs, cold packs, electrical stimulation, iontophoresis, and other similar direct applications to the skin are likely the mechanism leading to a burn of one's skin. From an overall healthcare perspective, burns have been identified as one of the most common injuries associated with physical therapy malpractice claims. From its own data, the Healthcare Providers Service Organization, which offers professional liability insurance to physical therapists, notes that burns contribute to 16.4% of all of their closed claims and that the average cost of a burn-related claim is $78,422 with severe burns resulting in a claim closer to $280,688.[15]

HPSO lists the most common causes of burns as improper use by the clinician, equipment failure or malfunction, and failure to properly supervise a patient. As an athletic trainer responsible for a large volume of athletes at any given time during treatment times, taping times, or any other busy scheduled rehabilitation period, one can easily relate to how proper supervision of even one person who has a hot pack or an iontophoresis unit applied that is not removed in a timely manner or if an athlete is asking for assistance because of the sensation not feeling right as in too hot from the hot pack or a burning/tingling sensation with any electrode directly on the skin.

From a legal perspective, keep in mind once again that a burn that results from negligence is not only associated with a physically noticeable scarring and/or disfigurement of one's superficial skin resulting in financial awards from a judge or jury. Some examples of legal action considerations following a burn resulting from malpractice may include the following:

- All associated medical expenses to include surgeries, rehabilitation, laboratories, medical imaging, etc.
- Payment for lost wages due to not being able to work to include future earning potential
- Payment for both physical and emotional pain and suffering

It is not the primary intent of this textbook to provide clinical guidance for athletic trainers. However, understanding how to mitigate risk is a key factor in preventing malpractice when it comes to burning a patient. For example, aside from assuring proper supervision at all times, the following should be considered as part of a harm reduction strategy:

- Be able to support your appropriate education and training to perform the task in accordance with the standard of care.
- Explain thoroughly what the procedure entails and what the patient should expect, proposed benefits, and potential risks, while then obtaining informed consent to perform the procedure.
- Properly expose and drape a patient so that only the necessary area of one's body is exposed and apply the pads/device to the target tissue.

- Perform a thorough assessment of the physical appearance and the dermatomal sensation of the area to be treated both prior to and at the completion of the application.
- Rule out any contradictions to an application including, but not limited to, decreased skin sensation, sensitivity to heat or cold, and open wounds not desirable to direct contact with a physical agent.
- Determine that all modes of application are in proper function condition, including clean pad adherence and calibration for electrical devices.
- Verify the temperature of an applied mode (hot or cold pack) falls within acceptable ranges.
- Document all aspects of the intervention, including photographs if necessary.

Here is an example of case law taking place in 2007 in the District Court of Appeal of the Second District of Florida cited as Corbo v. Garcia.[16] This case involves Christopher Corbo (physical therapist) and Precision Physical Therapy & Rehabilitation of Florida, PA v. Eulalia Garcia. The patient (plaintiff), Ms. Garcia claimed that Mr. Corbo failed to exercise reasonable and ordinary care in maintaining the electrical stimulation equipment used which resulted in burns to both of her arms. The courts noted that "the claimant shall have the burden of proving by the greater weight of evidence that the alleged actions of the health care provider represented a breach of the prevailing professional standard of care for that specific health care provider." In other words, the alleged injury was a direct result of the physical therapy treatment provided. If so, a wrongful act was the result of improper application of the device and/or the use of the physical therapist's professional judgment or skill. Part of this claim is that the physical therapist and/or company did not properly maintain the electrical stimulation equipment that is required in accordance with the expected standard of care. Regardless of the findings, one can see how many of the preventive steps previously described can bode well for avoiding this type of situation. As always, the claimant must prove all of the elements to find one negligent.

Another case can be summarized from the chiropractic profession in 2016.[17] Here, plaintiff Nicole Lawi, a patient, sued Daniel Fenster, a chiropractor affiliated with Complete Wellness Medical, P.C. claiming she suffered a permanent scar on her lower back related to a burn from Dr Fenster applying electrical stimulation as part of his treatment intervention. In this case, the plaintiff's expert chiropractic witness alleged that Dr Fenster departed from the standard of care by failing to properly perform the procedure with inadequate electrode pad preparation, and that as a result of the pads drying out from no use of gel contamination led to burning the patient's skin. Dr Fenster testified that he explained in detail the purpose of the treatment and what the patient should expect and also what not to expect. There were discrepancies as to whether the skin burn was the result of the electrodes or ice application afterward, as the plaintiff sought advice from friends of hers who are doctors. Again, here in this case, there is a burden on the plaintiff to prove that the chiropractor departed from the standard of care and as a result of doing so said harm was the result. Both parties had experts testify on their behalf, each presenting with different views. Of greatest interest is the fact that the defendant's expert testified that while the plaintiff did in fact experience a burn that resulted in a permanent scar on her back, the expert did not opine that such was a result of the omission or commission on the part of Dr Fenster. In other words, the evidence in this case does not support any causation. There are many more details to this case, yet one should be able to gather such facts that if you adhere to the standard of care on all fronts sometimes things simply happen and they are not in fact caused by something you did or did not do as an athletic trainer. Ultimately this case was dismissed based on the lack of clear causation and deviation from the standard of care when applying electrical stimulation.

Drug Testing

Drug testing in athletics is not new[18] and the underlying issue of conflict with the United States Constitution remains unchanged.[19] At a very basic level, drug testing equates to a search.

The Fourth Amendment of the Constitution clearly states the right of citizens to be protected from: "unreasonable searches and seizures shall not be violated, and no Warrants shall issue, but upon probable cause."[20]

The underlying issue with drug testing in athletics stems from the "probably cause" verbiage in the Fourth Amendment. Random, suspicionless drug test was a challenge in public schools in Vernonia v Acton.[21] In the Vernonia case a public school student challenged the school's requirement to comply with a drug testing protocol in order to participate in extracurricular activities. The case eventually progressed to the US Supreme Court where the desire of the school system to curtail illegal drug use was balanced with the rights of students.[22] The court compared the weight of creating and maintaining a safe environment for students to the rights of individual students. Ultimately, the court ruled in favor of the school system with Justice Anthony Scalia citing an "immediate and pressing' state interest on the part of the school in establishing the drug testing program.[22] It is important to remember that the constitutionality of random, suspicionless drug testing in a public school was upheld because the program was intended to protect the health of students. Drug testing in other arenas may or may not be primarily focused on participant health. In these circumstances, drug testing may be treated very differently by a court.

Drug testing in college athletics was initiated by the NCAA in 1994. Like drug testing in interscholastic athletics, the legality of drug testing in college athletics was challenged on the basis of it violating the Fourth Amendment of the Constitution.[23] Elizabeth O'Halloran was a student athlete at the University of Washington when she challenged the university drug testing program which was created and operated in compliance with NCAA guidelines and requirements. Although O'Halloran did not name the NCAA in the litigation she was, in a very real sense, placing the NCAA testing program under the scrutiny of the US Constitution. The case was ultimately decided in favor of the University. It must be noted that the interest of the NCAA in drug testing is two-fold. One objective is to protect the health of the student athlete. Without question, however, the second interest of the program is promoting fair competition, as evidenced by the extensive list of banned performance-enhancing drugs published by the NCAA. On an interesting side note, the relationship between the University of Washington and the NCAA, and the NCAA-mandated drug testing program is challenged with the NCAA being considered a third party to the litigation. The court stated that they would not address the relationship between the university and the NCAA and, in doing so, failed to clarify the issue of a state agent (the University of Washington) and a private actor (the NCAA) and the conflicting roles of each, unresolved.

Drug testing of Olympic athletes can get complicated and, at times, political.[24] Olympic athletes in the USA fall under the governance of the United States Olympic Committee. The authority of the USOC was clearly established by the Amateur Sports Act of 1978. While the history and political events behind the Amateur Sports Act are outside the scope of this text, the impact of being under the governance of the USOC, relative to drug testing, is not. The USOC signed a document known as the Olympic Charter. In doing so, the USOC, which governs all Olympic sport athletes in the USA, agreed to be governed and directed by the International Olympic Committee. A key element of that relationship is that Olympic athletes in the USA are expected to abide by the Olympic Charter and are asked to relinquish their right to resolving disputes, including those related to drug testing, through litigation.[25] Instead, Olympic athletes are expected to take drug-related eligibility issues to the Court of Arbitration of Sport, in Lausanne, Switzerland. Successfully challenging the authority of the USOC or the IOC through the US court system is rare, with most courts citing the establishment of the USOC as the single authority of Olympic sports and Olympic athletes in the USA.[26]

Professional athletes are not immune from drug testing. Congress took up the issue of mandating drug testing in professional sports but was unsuccessful.[27] Any drug testing program in a professional sport has to be approved through the collective bargaining agreement process. The players' association will have a great deal of influence on the outcome. Drug testing in professional sports is complicated by the bottom line: These are professional athletes and they are governed by their collective bargaining agreement.

Falls

One of the most common inadvertent injuries that occur and result in lawsuits is related to falls. In fact, it has been reported that falls compromise some 30.6% of all physical therapy professional liability closed claims.[28] Many athletic trainers work with generally younger aged athletes and do not assume that an injury from a general fall would be at the top of the list to consider in a risk management plan. However, falls in these populations can occur when one either is injured to the lower extremity or sustains an injury that interferes with their vision. Falls can occur as a result of a concussion that leads to balance disturbances. Falls can also simply occur when a surface is slippery. Each of these examples is the result of acts of omission that relate to inadequate supervision or ambulatory support, facility maintenance, or other causes. Additionally, more and more athletic trainers are working with an older yet physically active population that may have comorbidities that contribute to accidental falls.

In the physical therapy setting, failure to monitor or supervise a patient is reported as the top reason for most falls.[28] Of great interest is that in many of these cases the clinician is aware that the patient may be at some risk for falling, but has an established relationship with the patient as such as to provide only minimal assistance and supervision at best. For example, in an athletic training clinic, one might interpret this as having a line of sight on a person who had a recent knee surgery performing some standing exercises while the athletic trainer is taping ankles just 20 feet away.[29] Always keep in mind that similar to emergency action planning prior to a sporting event, having a plan, disseminating it to all stakeholders, and frequent education can play a critical role in minimizing falls. Furthermore, simply because someone does fall does not necessarily mean that the athletic trainer present or even not nearby is held negligent.

Some simple yet important steps an athletic trainer should take with every patient to minimize the risk of a fall may include the following:

- Perform an adequate assessment of one's risk for falling (balance, strength, etc.)
- Screen for any cognitive issues that may impair one's recall of safety measures
- Deliver detailed yet layperson education regarding fall prevention
- Check assistive devices, furniture, flooring, and rails for proper function
- Observe patient transfer, walk, safely use assistive devices, navigate steps, etc.
- Complete timely and thorough documentation each session

Supervision

As previously noted, proper supervision is always reviewed at the heart of any lawsuit, and in many cases, the lack thereof plays some role that questions negligence on the part of the clinician. Not providing proper supervision and/or adhering to one's legal supervisory scope of practice is an act of omission. Here are some thoughts to consider related to the many aspects of supervision in the athletic training profession:

Athletic Trainer to Patient Supervision: In all settings, athletic trainers must establish clear definitions of supervision as it relates to individual patients as well as a group of athletes. In order to demonstrate and justify a responsibility of care, one must determine in all situations if appropriate supervision is being met. Each of the following examples should be supported with written documentation that is disseminated and adhered to at all times.

Athletic Trainer to Aide/Intern Supervision: While there may not be a legal definition for this on a statewide basis or as it relates to professional standards, anyone serving in a non-licensed and non-academic role will have significant restrictions on the tasks that they are allowed to perform. The obvious limitations may be on clinical interventions, but it is important to be cognizant of the fact that even if an intern or an aide is responsible for cleaning tables and/or floor surfaces, an ultimate slip and fall or acquired skin conditions from the environment may come back to the evidence of how such an individual was trained and supervised by the licensed athletic trainer.

Athletic Trainer Preceptor to Student Supervision: This relationship can be defined by academic standards and/or state licensure guidelines. Regardless, an athletic training preceptor must determine the proper guidelines for the supervision of an athletic training student formally enrolled in a CAATE-accredited program. This becomes a challenge as one might personally decide that based on different students' levels of knowledge, experience, and professionalism that the level and type of supervision may vary. In fact the level of supervision may change over the course of time that a student is with a preceptor. Regardless, adhering to guidelines that assure proper supervision is essential.

Aide/Intern/Student to Patient Supervision: Non-licensed personnel working under the supervision of an athletic trainer will have limited allowable tasks to perform. Yet, interactions with patients ranging from communication exchanges to observation can play a very important role in a patient's outcome. All tasks should be made extremely clear, placed in writing, and signed off by all parties.

Athletic Trainer/Physician Supervision/Direction: Standard 1 of the Board of Certification Practice Standards reads as follows: "Direction: The athletic trainer renders service or treatment under the direction of, or in collaboration with a physician, in accordance with their training and the state's statutes, rules and regulations."[30] This alone is essential to have a policy and written updated standing orders for. Furthermore, Standard 15 of the CAATE guidelines reads as follows: "Standard 15: Describe the methods used to ensure that the athletic training and/or supplemental clinical experience and the style of preceptor supervision and feedback are developmentally appropriate for each student based on his/her progression in the program." Within the same guidelines the glossary defines the term supervision as follows:

Supervision occurs along a developmental continuum that allows a student to move from interdependence to independence based on the student's knowledge and skills as well as the context of care. Preceptors must be onsite and have the ability to intervene on behalf of the athletic training student and the patient. Supervision also must occur in compliance with the state practice act of the state in which the student is engaging in client/patient care. If the patient/client care is occurring via telehealth or telemedicine, the preceptor must concurrently monitor the patient/client care through appropriate telecommunication technology.[30]

As an example, in the state of Florida, under the athletic training scope of practice Rule No. 64B33–4.001 "direction," athletic trainers must practice under the supervision of a physician licensed under chapters 458, 459, or 460, or otherwise authorized by Florida law to practice medicine. The physician can provide direction through written or oral protocols or prescriptions, and the athletic trainer must provide care and service as directed.[31]

Nohr summarizes a 2011 decision[32] from a Federal Court in Alabama of a former Auburn University football player who sued an athletic trainer at the University for failing to supervise his rehabilitation appropriately. The plaintiff claims to have gotten injured while performing weight training activities directed by the athletic trainer that were not in order with the physician's timetable and therefore unsafe to perform. As a result of a subsequent injury, the player was unable to continue his football career and his scholarship was terminated. The case was dismissed because the court was unable to prove that the conduct of the athletic trainer caused the player's injury. However, you can see here how the relationship between the athletic trainer and physician, as well as the athletic trainer and athlete, plays into the definition of supervision.

References

1. Tahoma Schools Settle with Teen in Football-injury Case. *The Seattle Times.* September 17, 2009. Accessed October 30, 2024. https://www.seattletimes.com/seattle-news/tahoma-schools-settle-with-teen-in-football-injury-case/
2. *Concussion Legislation by State.* Accessed October 30, 2024. https://convention.shapeamerica.org/Convention/standards/guidelines/Concussion/state-policy.aspx
3. SSI_ARRINGTONSETTLEMENTAGREEMENT.pdf. Accessed October 30, 2024. https://ncaaorg.s3.amazonaws.com/ssi/concussion/SSI_ARRINGTONSETTLEMEN-TAGREEMENT.pdf
4. Laskas JM. The Brain That Sparked the NFL's Concussion Crisis. *The Atlantic.* December 2, 2015. Accessed October 31, 2024. https://www.theatlantic.com/health/archive/2015/12/the-nfl-players-brain-that-changed-the-history-of-the-concussion/417597/
5. Owens D, Solomon K. *In the United States District Court for the Northern District of Illinois Eastern Division.* 2015. The U.S. District Court for the Northern District of Illinois.
6. *Reports & Statistics.* Accessed October 31, 2024. https://www.nflconcussionsettlement.com/Reports_Statistics.aspx
7. Kucera KL, Colgate B, Cantu RC. *Annual Survey of Football Injury Research.* Published online 2023. https://nccsir.unc.edu/wp-content/uploads/sites/5614/2024/02/Annual-Football-2023-Fatalities-FINAL-WEB.pdf
8. National Athletic Trainers Association. *The Inter-association Task Force on Exertional Heat-Illness.* June 2003. Accessed October 30, 2024. Heat Illness Consensus Statement
9. *Stringer v. Minnesota Vikings*, 705 N.W.2d 746 (2005)
10. *Launch of the Korey Stringer Institute.* Accessed October 30, 2024. https://youtu.be/MeQJupxI7fs
11. Henry D, Sachs K, Hodge DP. *Pushing Players Too Far to "Do Something" Will Not "Win the Day" in Court—Takeaways from Two UO Suits.* Published online 2019. https://www.mmwr.com/pushing-players-too-far-to-do-something-will-not-win-the-day-in-court-takeaways-from-two-uo-suits/
12. Meier DT. *Primary Assumption of Risk and Duty in Football Indirect Injury Cases: A Legal Workout from the Tragedies on the Training Ground for American Values.* 2002. https://heinonline.org/HOL/LandingPage?handle=hein.journals/virspelj2&div=3&id=&page=
13. *Stowers v. Clay City Central School Corp.*, 855 N.E.2d.739 (2006)
14. Walters, R. *Walters Report to USM Board of Regents.* Walters, Inc.; September 21, 2018.
15. Healthcare Providers Service Organization. *Risk Management Spotlight: Burns.* Fort Washington, PA: HPSO; 2020.

16. *Corbo v. Garcia.*, 949 So. 2d. 366 (Fla. Dist. Ct. App.) 2007
17. *Lawi v. Complete Wellness Med.*, P.C., 2020 N.Y Slip Op. 33659 Decided October 28, 2020
18. National Collegiate Athletic Association. *NCAA Drug Testing.* Updated 2024. Accessed October 30, 2024. NCAA Drug Testing Program - NCAA.org
19. Cranford, M. Drug Testing and the Right to Privacy: Arguing the Ethics of Workplace Drug Testing. *Journal of Business Ethics.* 1998;17(16):1805–1815.
20. Pommett, FA. Recent Developments: Vernonia School District 47KJ v. Acton. *University of Baltimore Law Forum.* 1996;26(2).
21. Shutler, SE. Random, Suspicion-less Drug Testing of High School Athletes. *The Journal of Criminal Law and Criminology.* 1996;86(4).
22. *Vernonia School District v. Acton*, 515 U.S. 646 (1995)
23. *O'Halloran v. University of Washington*, 679 F. Supp. 997 (W.D. Wash. 1988)
24. National Public Radio. Let's Talk about China's Whopping Olympic Medal Count. August 2, 2024. Accessed October 30, 2024. 2024 Paris Olympics: NPR.
25. *Michels v. United States Olympic Committee*, 2020 N.Y. Slip Op. 33659. Decided October 28, 2020.
26. Cox TW. The International War against Doping: Limiting the Collateral Damage from Strict Liability. *Vanderbilt Law Review.* 2021;47:295. https://scholarship.law.vanderbilt.edu/vjtl/vol47/iss1/5
27. ESPN. *U.S. Pro Sports Leagues Still Trail in Drug-testing Arms Race.* Updated May 22, 2008. Accessed October 30, 2024. ESPN - Serving Sports Fans. Anytime. Anywhere.
28. Healthcare Providers Service Organization. *Risk Management Spotlight: Home Care Final.* Fort Washington, PA: HPSO; 2020.
29. Perspective _ 5 Ways the CDC Guidance Shows How Physical Therapy Is Leading the Way in Post-COVID-19 Care. *APTA.html.*
30. NATA Board of Certification, Inc. *BOC Standards of Professional Practice.* December 2023. Accessed October 30, 2024. SOPP-2024.pdf
31. Florida Department of Health. Florida Administrative Code and Florida Administrative Register. *Standard of Practice, Board of Athletic Training.* January 6, 2006, 64B33–4.001: Protocols; Scope of Practice - Florida Administrative Rules, Law, Code, Register - FAC, FAR, eRulemaking
32. SportsRisk: Solutions in Recreation Risk Management. *Athletic Trainer Risk Management. Nohr, KM.* January 17, 2017. Accessed October 30, 2024. Risk Management Newsletter | SportRisk

9 Discrimination

Chapter Objectives: Following the completion of this chapter, the reader will:

1. Define and differentiate between key terms related to diversity, equity, and inclusion
2. Identify the impact of landmark court rulings related to gender/sex discrimination, racial/ethnicity discrimination, discrimination of the LGBTQIA+ community, and discrimination of those with disabilities
3. Analyze strategies and best practices to mitigate discrimination to foster a more inclusive and equitable practice

Introduction

In the current sociopolitical climate in the United States, discussions about equity, diversity, and inclusion are hotly debated and often politically charged. While these principles are neither new nor novel, there has been an intentional shift in healthcare to highlight the impact of these inequities in the communities served. For example, the Quintuple Aim as put forth by the Institute for Healthcare Improvement (IHI) seeks to optimize healthcare system performance through improved patient experiences and elevate the importance of and impact of health equity. Furthermore, the components directly address the impact of the social determinants of health and inequities in the healthcare system[1] while placing an intentional focus on the reduction of health disparities[2]. Within the profession of athletic training, the core components of equity, compassion, and respecting the dignity of others form the backbone of the NATA Code of Ethics[3] and the BOC Code of Professional Responsibility[4]. Additionally, the 2020 Commission on Accreditation of Athletic Training Education (CAATE) standards require programs to document how they integrate and assess DEI principles in curriculum development and delivery[5].

It is important to recognize that health inequities affect diverse populations that extend beyond race and gender. Patients from rural communities, patients of differing socioeconomic status, patients with varying levels of ability/disability, and those that identify within the LGBTQIA+ community are all at higher risk for experiencing health inequities[6]. Furthermore, patients with intersecting identities

DOI: 10.4324/9781003524823-9

are at an even greater risk of experiencing these imbalances in access, treatment, and positive health outcomes[7].

The remainder of this chapter focuses on specific examples of discrimination and discriminatory practices. While many of the hallmark cases discussed are not directly related to athletic training, they were intentionally chosen to highlight the most prevalent forms of discrimination in healthcare while providing historical and conceptual context to contemporary legal statutes.

Gender- and Sex-Based Discrimination

Gender, as defined by the APA Dictionary of Psychology, is "the socially constructed roles, behaviors, activities, and attributes that a given society considers appropriate for different genders"[8]. This differs from the term sex, which is related to biological attributes of being male, female, or intersex[9]. Examples of gender- and sex-based discrimination can include, but are not limited to, sexual harassment, discrimination based on sexual orientation, refusing to hire a candidate after learning their gender identity, repeated and purposefully misgendering or mispronouncing an individual, and refusing an employee to use the restroom associated with the gender the employee identifies with[10].

Gender- and sex-based discrimination cases are unfortunately neither new nor unique to healthcare and specifically the profession of athletic training. A 2015 study by Bruce et al. found that 87% of female surgical residents encountered some form of gender-based discrimination in medical school, 88% reported gender-based discrimination in residency, and 91% reported gender-based discrimination in clinical practice[11]. These statistics are echoed in a 2020 study of physicians by Lu et al. which found that nearly 53% of female respondents reported unwanted sexual behaviors in their careers (compared to 26% of male respondents) and approximately 63% of female faculty respondents reported experiences of gender-based discrimination (compared to 12% of male faculty respondents)[12]. The data are just as staggering for gender- and sex-based discrimination in athletic training. A 2022 study by Trentley et al. examined the experiences of professional masters' athletic training students and their experiences with sexual harassment. The authors reported that 35% of female respondents reported being subjected to sexual harassment (compared to 5% of male respondents)[13]. Previous studies on sexual harassment in athletic training found that 64% of female respondents had been sexually harassed at some point in their educational or professional careers.[14]

Title IX

One of the most influential pieces of legislation related to gender- and sex-based discrimination has been the passage and evolution of Title IX. Originally passed in 1972, Title IX bars sex-based discrimination in educational programs and activities offered that receive federal funding.[15] Prior to its passage, women were often excluded or had limited access to educational programs, had limited access to scholarships, and were held to different admissions standards compared to their male counterparts. Additionally, female faculty were denied tenure more frequently compared to their

male counterparts[16]. Since the passage of Title IX, the percentage of female enrollment in higher education has increased at a greater rate than male enrollment leading to a tripling of the percentage of women aged 25–34 with a college degree[17]. In
1975, President Nixon signed the Title IX athletics regulations, which guaranteed that
women and men would have equitable opportunities to participate in sports. These
regulations also provide allotted scholarships to women and men that are proportional
to their participation in sport. Furthermore, women and men are provided with equal
treatment related to other benefits, including equipment, supplies, practice/travel
schedules, per diem, and access to benefits such as tutoring and medical care.[18] Cases
such as *Cohen v. Brown University*[19, 20] (1996), *Biediger v. Quinnipiac University*[21]
(2012), and *Communities for Equity v. Michigan High School Athletic Association*[22]
(2001) provided expansion opportunities for women to equally participate in sports
while also ensuring schools provided equal treatment for women's and men's sports.

The outcome of the *Cohen* case still has real-world implications for Brown's athletic department. In May 2020, the university announced that it would discontinue
six women's varsity and five men's varsity sports, including men's cross country and
track and field, stating that these sports were specifically chosen to remain compliant with the 1998 settlement agreement. However, the university would ultimately
reverse their decision to discontinue men's track and field and cross country. Considering this reversal, a motion was filed by female student athletes at Brown to enforce
the original 1998 ruling. As a result, the university agreed to a settlement that rein-
stated and restored two women's teams to varsity status, agreed to not add any additional men's varsity programs, and that if any men's teams were to be reconsidered
to be elevated to varsity status, two additional women's teams would be elevated to
varsity status. While the terms of this agreement remained in effect until August 31,
2024, the university must still comply with federal Title IX provisions.[19, 20]

Over the last 30 years, additional amendments and cases have shaped the application of Title IX provisions in education. The cases of *Gebser v. Lago Vista Independent School District*[23] (1998) and *Davis v. Monroe County Board of Education*[24] (1999)
helped to establish the need for schools to provide safe environments for students and
to address sexual harassment of students by their peers or teachers. The *Putman v.
Board of Education of Somerset Independent School*[25] (2000) case reaffirmed that the
provisions outlined in Title IX regulations prohibit sexual harassment and discrimination based on gender stereotypes based on actual or perceived sexual orientation, and
Lopez v. Metropolitan Government of Nashville[26] (2010) secured protections against
sexual harassment and assault against students with disabilities. Additional cases of
gender- and sex-based discrimination specifically affecting the LGBTQIA+ community are addressed in a later portion of this chapter.

Racial and Ethnic Discrimination

As with the concept of gender, race and ethnicity are social constructs that are
utilized to categorize groups of individuals. Whereas race categorizes individuals
based on shared physical traits and biological attributes[27] (i.e., White/Caucasian,
Black/African American, Hispanic/Latino, Asian American, and Native American),
ethnicity classifies individuals based on having a shared culture, customs/traditions,
language, values, and beliefs[28] (i.e., Italian, German, Jordanian, and Chinese).
Similarly to gender and sex, race and ethnicity are often used interchangeably.

Like the gender- and sex-based discrimination cases previously discussed, racial and ethnic discrimination cases are also unfortunately neither new nor unique to healthcare. While efforts are being made to actively recruit and retain healthcare providers of color[29–32], data show that these groups of providers remain significantly underrepresented compared to their white counterparts. According to the 2019 data from the Association of American Medical Colleges, 56% of the active physician workforce identified as white as compared to 17% that identify as Asian, 6% that identify as Hispanic, and 5% that identify as Black[33]. A 2019 systematic review by Snyder and Schwartz[34] found that healthcare providers of color faced racial discrimination in the workplace reported greater dissatisfaction in their careers and greater disparate career outcomes than their white counterparts. In athletic training, the data are more staggering with 80% of NATA members identifying as white, 6% identifying as Hispanic, 4% identifying as Black, and 4% identifying as Asian.[35] Similar to the study by Snyder and Schwartz, a 2024 article by Smith et al.[36] found that newly certified athletic trainers of color reported the presence of microaggressions in the workplace to include inappropriate racial comments and actions, as well as an overall lack of support in their educational training and transition to clinical practice.

However, even with the protections outlined in Title VII of the Civil Rights Act of 1964[37] and the establishment of the Equal Employment Opportunity Commission (EEOC), high-profile cases involving racial and ethnic discrimination have become more prevalent and more frequent over the last decade. The murder of George Floyd and subsequent trial, the cases involving Breonna Taylor and Elijah McClain, the increase in hate crimes directed against Asian Americans during the COVID-19 pandemic, and the rise in antisemitic speech have become a mainstay in the American media and across social media platforms. A 2022 publication from the Anti-Defamation League reported the highest rate on record of documented reports of antisemitic harassment, violence, and vandalism[38], with a 2024 report from the Anti-Defamation League highlighting the uptick in antisemitic speech following the October 7, 2023 Hamas terror attack.[39] The prevalence of these high-profile incidents continues to illustrate the complexity of both the impact and limitations of judicial rulings in addressing systemic inequality.

Discrimination of the LGBTQ+ Community

As with gender/sex and race/ethnicity, it is important to understand the appropriate terminology as it applies to members of the LGBTQIA+ community. The Center of Excellence on LGBTQ+ Behavioral Health Equity has developed a robust list of terms and definitions related to sexual orientation, gender identity, and expression (SOGIE)[40]. Specifically created for athletic trainers, the National Athletic Trainers' Association (NATA) LGBTQIA+ Advisory Committee has developed and procured resources for its members to help clinicians effectively treat the diverse needs of these patients. This comprehensive collection of resources can be helpful for athletic trainers and other healthcare providers to understand the growing needs of this diverse patient population and includes strategies for incorporating best practices for inclusive healthcare.[41]

Similarly to the cases presented in the previous sections, discrimination cases involving the LGBTQIA+ community have become more public facing over the last decade.[42] Hate crimes against the LGBTQIA+ community rose by more than 19% in 2022[43], and the percentage goes up exponentially in states that have anti-LGBTQIA+ laws, especially on K-12 campuses[44]. According to the Human Rights Campaign, in 2023 there were over 520 anti-LGBTQIA+ bills that were introduced at the state level and over 200 bills specifically targeting anti-transgender and non-binary people.[45] Since 2020, 25 states have passed laws restricting transgender athletes' abilities to participate in sports.[46] Additionally, the US House of Representatives passed *HR734 Protection of Women and Girls in Sports Act of 2023*[47] which would not allow transwomen (an individual assigned male at birth) from competing in programs that are meant for women and girls. Furthermore, at the time of print, 18 states currently have laws that ban transgender athletes from competing in school sports, with Oklahoma being the only state that requires a signed affidavit to attest to a student's assigned sex[48]. It is vital for athletic trainers and healthcare providers to stay informed about these legislative matters to fully understand and address their profound impact on LGBTQIA+ patients' health and well-being.

Disability and Ableism

One aspect of discrimination that often goes overlooked is that of differing levels of ability. Disability, as defined by the APA Dictionary of Psychology, is "a lasting physical or mental impairment that significantly interferes with an individual's ability to function in one or more central life activities, such as self-care, ambulation, communication, social interaction, sexual expression, or employment."[49] As such, ableism is a type of discrimination that favors those who are able-bodied and without disability. A 2022 systematic review by Lindsay et al.[50] examined the experiences and impact of workplace discrimination and ableism in healthcare providers over the last 20 years. The authors found that discrimination and ableism occurred at both the institutional and individual levels and found a lack of reporting of discrimination due to fear, stigma, and retribution on career development and advancement.[50] While we predominantly consider disability categories such as visual, auditory, mental, and physical, conditions such as cancer, diabetes, major depressive disorder, and post-traumatic stress disorder can also be considered a disability by law.

The Americans with Disabilities Act (ADA)[51] became law in 1990 and sought to prohibit discrimination against individuals with disabilities in areas of public and private life, and to ensure that those with disabilities have the same rights and protections as those without disabilities. As with the provisions outlined in Title VII of the Civil Rights Act, Title I of the ADA ensures that people with disabilities have equal access to employment opportunities. Additionally, Title III of the ADA ensures that public buildings (within the 12 defined categories set by the ADA) are accessible to those with disabilities and ensures that new construction is compliant with ADA standards. In addition to the passage of the ADA, several cases have championed the rights of athletes with disabilities. In *PGA Tour Inc. v. Martin*[52] *(2001)*, the Supreme Court ruled in favor of a player's request for accommodations to use a golf cart due to their degenerative medical condition. More recently, in the case of *Urso v. Team Illinois, Inc*[53](2024), the courts ruled that sports teams could not discriminate against their players. In this instance, the athlete disclosed her history of anxiety and depression to her coach and was subsequently kicked off the team.

Strategies to Mitigate Discriminatory Practices

To begin to address change to impact these complex issues outlined in this chapter, it is essential for healthcare providers to implement a range of comprehensive mitigation strategies aimed at promoting more inclusive, accessible, and equitable patient-centered care. The strategies outlined subsequently provide a starting point for clinicians to utilize within their own practice and reflect the first steps in dismantling these inequities.

Engage in ongoing cultural competency training: It is imperative that providers integrate and actively engage in ongoing cultural competency training that is aimed at increasing awareness of personal and professional biases. These trainings should address diversity in patient populations that extend beyond traditional racial and gender differences, with an intentional focus placed on how delivery of care may need to be adjusted to meet diverse patient needs. Research shows that these trainings have a positive impact on enhanced clinical outcomes, improved patient satisfaction, and improved the knowledge, attitudes, and skills of the provider.[54-56] Furthermore, these trainings could have an effect on decreasing health disparities through fostering better communication between provider and patient, thereby enhancing patient trust and improving the patient experience.[54-56]

Create and foster an inclusive facility: The NATA LGBTQ+ Advisory Committee has created numerous resources for athletic trainers to help in the creation of an inclusive facility for all patients. Resources such as ways to develop more inclusive policies and procedures, strategies to update medical documents, and other information can be found on the NATA website[41].

Foster a diverse workforce through recruitment and retention efforts: As previously mentioned, there is currently an intentional focus in healthcare to recruit and retain providers of color[29-32]. However, efforts must also be made to recruit and retain providers from additional diverse backgrounds (i.e., gender, level of ability, sexual orientation, and socioeconomic status) to truly ensure an inclusive healthcare system designed to meet diverse patient needs. Additionally, employers engaged in the hiring process should broaden their recruitment efforts by advertising on platforms that cater to diverse and underrepresented communities.

Incorporation of health equity and cultural competency into medical curriculum: As previously mentioned, the current iteration of the 2020 Commission on Accreditation of Athletic Training Education (CAATE) standards specifically requires documentation of how programs are incorporating and assessing DEI principles in their program development and delivery of curricular content[5]. These types of standards can also be found in medical school[57], physical therapy education[58], and nursing education[59] to name a few. Content including the impact of the social determinants of health, adverse childhood events, historical health inequities, and discussion of marginalized and underrepresented communities can be helpful in fostering a new generation of culturally sensitive providers.

Conclusion

Although progress has been made in addressing some of the discriminatory practices discussed, work remains to achieve a truly equitable and inclusive society. The historical cases presented continue to have relevance today by providing the framework to understand the systemic barriers that still affect our communities. By examining how these cases have shaped contemporary healthcare practices and our sociopolitical landscape, providers can recognize that disparities still exist and use this knowledge to take meaningful steps toward enacting change.

CASE STUDY ACTIVITY

Case Study #1: Laura is an athletic trainer applying for a head athletic trainer position at a major Division I university. She has over 15 years of experience and was previously the head athletic trainer at a different university. During the interview process, she meets with Michael, the athletic director, who repeatedly questions her ability in being able to work with male athletes and how she will "handle" working with the head football coach. Ultimately, Michael decides not to hire Laura and chooses to hire Chris, a less-experienced male candidate, for the job.

Questions:

1. Does Laura have a case for discrimination? Why or why not?
2. How might Michael's assumptions about Laura's capabilities be reflective of greater biases about gender roles in society and athletics?
3. What legal cases and additional resources could Laura use to support her case of discrimination? Why?

Case Study #2: Ashley, a Black female athletic trainer, has been working at a professional sports team for five years. Despite her experience and consistently positive evaluations, she has been passed over for promotion several times in favor of her white male colleagues. She has noticed that her contributions and suggestions are often downplayed or ignored in meetings, and her requests for additional leadership roles and training have been ignored or denied.

1. Does Ashley have grounds for a discrimination case? Why or why not?
2. How do Ashley's experiences reflect the intersectionality of race and gender discrimination in the workplace?
3. What steps could Ashley's workplace take in order to ensure compliance with anti-discriminatory policies?

References

1. Farrell TW, Greer AG, Bennie S, Hageman H, Pfeifle A. Academic Health Centers and the Quintuple Aim of Health Care. *Academic Medicine*. 2023;98(5). https://journals.lww.com/academicmedicine/fulltext/2023/05000/academic_health_centers_and_the_quintuple_aim_of.24.aspx

2. Nundy S, Cooper LA, Mate KS. The Quintuple Aim for Health Care Improvement: A New Imperative to Advance Health Equity. *JAMA*. 2022;327(6):521–522. doi:10.1001/jama.2021.25181

3. National Athletic Trainers' Association. *Code of Ethics*. Published online 2002. Accessed October 6, 2024. https://www.nata.org/sites/default/files/nata_code_of_ethics_2022.pdf

4. Board of Certification for the Athletic Trainer. *BOC Standards of Professional Practice*. Published online 2023. Accessed October 6, 2024. https://bocatc.org/wp-content/uploads/2024/01/SOPP−2024.pdf

5. Commission on Accreditation of Athletic Training Education. *Standards and Procedures for Accreditation of Professional Programs in Athletic Training*. 2024. Accessed October 6, 2024. https://caate.net/Portals/0/Standards_and_Procedures_Professional_Programs.pdf?ver=01iHqzdBAW0IsGARUc-19Q%3d%3d

6. Health Equity in Healthy People 2030 - Healthy People 2030. *health.gov*. Accessed October 6, 2024. https://health.gov/healthypeople/priority-areas/health-equity-healthy-people-2030

7. Pérez-Stable EJ, Webb Hooper M. The Pillars of Health Disparities Science—Race, Ethnicity, and Socioeconomic Status. *JAMA Health Forum*. 2023;4(12):e234463–e234463. doi:10.1001/jamahealthforum.2023.4463

8. Gender. In: *American Psychological Association*. https://dictionary.apa.org/gender

9. Sex. In: *American Psychological Association*. https://dictionary.apa.org/sex

10. US Equal Employment Opportunity Commission. *Sex Discrimination FAQs*. Accessed October 6, 2024. https://www.eeoc.gov/youth/sex-discrimination-faqs#:~:text=Examples%20of%20gender%20identity%20discrimination,to%20transition%2C%20or%20requiring%20employees

11. Bruce AN, Battista A, Plankey MW, Johnson LB, Marshall MB. Perceptions of Gender-based Discrimination during Surgical Training and Practice. *Medical Education Online*. 2015;20(1):25923. doi:10.3402/meo.v20.25923

12. Lu DW, Lall MD, Mitzman J, et al. #MeToo in EM: A Multicenter Survey of Academic Emergency Medicine Faculty on Their Experiences with Gender Discrimination and Sexual Harassment. *Western Journal of Emergency Medicine*. 2020;21(2):252–260. doi:10.5811/westjem.2019.11.44592

13. Trentley C, Bradney D, Singe S, Bowman T. The Experiences of Professional Master's Athletic Training Students with Sexual Harassment During Clinical Education. *Athletic Training Education Journal*. 2022;17:293–301. doi:10.4085/1947-380X-21-052

14. Shingles RR, Smith Y. Perceptions of Sexual Harassment in Athletic Training. *Athletic Training Education Journal*. 2008;3(3):102–107. doi:10.4085/1947-380X-3.3.102

15. Rights (OCR) O for C. Title IX of the Education Amendments of 1972. October 17, 2019. Accessed October 6, 2024. https://www.hhs.gov/civil-rights/for-individuals/sex-discrimination/title-ix-education-amendments/index.html

16. *Equal Access to Education: Forty Years of Title IX*. Published online June 23, 2012. https://www.justice.gov/sites/default/files/crt/legacy/2012/06/20/titleixreport.pdf

17. U.S. Department of Commerce. *Women in America: Indicators of Social and Economic Well-Being*. Published online March 2011. https://www2.census.gov/library/publications/2011/demo/womeninamerica.pdf

18. Title IX Frequently Asked Questions. *NCAA.org*. Accessed October 6, 2024. https://www.ncaa.org/sports/2014/1/27/title-ix-frequently-asked-questions.aspx

19. *Cohen v. Brown University* (United States District Court 1995). https://law.justia.com/cases/federal/district-courts/FSupp/879/185/2264922/

20. *Cohen v. Brown University* 1:92-cv-00197 (D.R.I.) | Civil Rights Litigation Clearing-house. Accessed October 6, 2024. https://clearinghouse.net/case/13910/

21. *Biediger v. Quinnipiac University* (Second Circuit 2012). https://law.justia.com/cases/federal/appellate-courts/ca2/10-3302/10-3302-2012-08-07.html

22. *Communities for Equity v. Michigan High School Athletic Association.* (United States District Court, W.D. Michigan, Southern Division 2001). https://law.justia.com/cases/federal/district-courts/FSupp2/178/805/2510014/

23. *Gebser v. Lago Vista Independent School Dist.* (Supreme Court 1998). https://supreme.justia.com/cases/federal/us/524/274/#top

24. *Davis v. Monroe County Board of Education.* (Supreme Court 1999). Accessed October 6, 2024. https://supreme.justia.com/cases/federal/us/526/629/

25. Civil Rights Division | Putman v. Board of Education of Somerset Ind. Schools. *Amicus Brief.* August 6, 2015. Accessed October 6, 2024. https://www.justice.gov/crt/putman-v-board-education-somerset-ind-schools-amicus-brief

26. *Lopez v. Metropolitan Government of Nashville.* (United States District Court 2009). https://law.justia.com/cases/federal/district-courts/tennessee/tnmdce/3:2007cv00799/39705/140/

27. Race. In: *APA Dictionary of Psychology.* Accessed October 6, 2024. https://dictionary.apa.org/

28. Ethnicity. In: *APA Dictionary of Psychology.* Accessed October 6, 2024. https://dictionary.apa.org/

29. Durkee MI. How to Recruit and Retain Faculty Members of Colour in Academia. *Nature Reviews Psychology.* 2022;1(9):489-490. doi:10.1038/s44159-022-00098-0

30. Baez S, Harris N. Inclusive Steps for Paving the Path for Racial and Ethnic Diversity in Athletic Training Research. *Journal of Athletic Training.* 2024;59(4):335–337. doi:10.4085/1062-6050-0315.23

31. Smith TY. The Time Is Now: A Model for Diversity Recruitment and Retention in Emergency Medicine Training Programs. *AEM Education and Training.* 2021;5(Suppl 1):S126-S129. doi:10.1002/aet2.10659

32. Adams WM, Terranova AB, Belval LN. Addressing Diversity, Equity, and Inclusion in Athletic Training: Shifting the Focus to Athletic Training Education. *Journal of Athletic Training.* 2021;56(2):129–133. doi:10.4085/1062-6050-0558-20

33. Diversity in Medicine: Facts and Figures 2019. *AAMC.* Accessed October 6, 2024. https://www.aamc.org/data-reports/workforce/report/diversity-medicine-facts-and-figures-2019

34. Snyder CR, Schwartz MR. Experiences of Workplace Racial Discrimination among People of Color in Healthcare Professions. *Journal of Cultural Diversity.* 2019; 26(3):96–107.

35. *Examining Ethnic Diversity in Athletic Training: NATA Leadership Report.* https://www.nata.org/sites/default/files/edac_leadership_diversity_report_2023.pdf

36. Smith AD, Moffit DM, Lacayo CP, Bowman TG. Challenges Faced during Professional Preparation and Transition to Practice among Diverse Early Professional Athletic Trainers. *Journal of Athletic Training.* 2024;59(5):536–545. doi:10.4085/1062-6050-0376.23

37. Title VII of the Civil Rights Act of 1964. *US EEOC.* Accessed October 6, 2024. https://www.eeoc.gov/statutes/title-vii-civil-rights-act-1964

38. Audit of Antisemitic Incidents. *ADL. Anti-Defamation League.* Accessed October 6, 2024. https://www.adl.org/audit-antisemitic-incidents

39. One Year Later: Antisemitic Trends Post-10/7. *ADL. Anti-Defamation League.* Accessed October 6, 2024. https://www.adl.org/resources/report/one-year-later-antisemitic-trends-post-107

40. Sexual Orientation, Gender Identity, & Expression Glossary of Terms. *Center of Excellence: LGBTQ+ Behavioral Health Equity.* Accessed October 6, 2024. https://lgbtqequity.org/wp-content/uploads/2023/04/SOGIE-Glossary-4.23.pdf

41. Resources. *NATA.* December 10, 2018. Accessed October 6, 2024. https://www.nata.org/professional-interests/inclusion/resources

42. Examples of Court Decisions Supporting Coverage of LGBT-Related Discrimination Under Title VII. *US EEOC*. Accessed October 6, 2024. https://www.eeoc.gov/
wysk/examples-court-decisions-supporting-coverage-lgbt-related-discrimination-
under-title-vii

43. *FBI Crime Statistics Show Anti-LGBTQ Hate Crimes on the Rise*. Accessed October 6,
2024. https://thehill.com/homenews/lgbtq/4259292-fbi-crime-statistics-show-anti-lgbt
q-hate-crimes-on-the-rise/

44. Meckler L, Natanson H, Harden JD. In States with Laws Targeting LGBTQ Issues,
School Hate Crimes Quadrupled. *Washington Post*. March 12, 2024. Accessed
October 6, 2024. https://www.washingtonpost.com/education/2024/03/12/school-lgbtq-
hate-crimes-incidents/.

45. Roundup of Anti-LGBTQ+ Legislation Advancing in States across the Country.
HRC. May 23, 2023. Accessed October 6, 2024. https://www.hrc.org/press-releases/
roundup-of-anti-lgbtq-legislation-advancing-in-states-across-the-country

46. *Movement Advancement Project | Bans on Transgender Youth Participation in Sports*.
Accessed October 7, 2024. https://www.lgbtmap.org/equality-maps/youth/sports_
participation_bans

47. Rep. Steube WG [R F 17. H.R.734 - 118th Congress (2023–2024): Protection of Women
and Girls in Sports Act of 2023. April 25, 2023. Accessed October 6, 2024. https://www.
congress.gov/bill/118th-congress/house-bill/734

48. Oklahoma Schools Now Require "Biological Sex Affidavit" for Student Athletes. *NBC News*. July 29, 2022. Accessed October 31, 2024. https://www.nbcnews.
com/nbc-out/out-politics-and-policy/oklahoma-schools-now-require-biological-
sex-affidavit-student-athletes-rcna40705

49. Disability. In: *APA Dictionary of Psychology*. Accessed October 6, 2024. https://diction-
ary.apa.org/

50. Lindsay S, Fuentes K, Ragunathan S, Lamaj L, Dyson J. Ableism within Health
Care Professions: A Systematic Review of the Experiences and Impact of Discrimination against Health Care Providers with Disabilities. *Disability and Rehabilitation*.
2023;45(17):2715–2731. doi:10.1080/09638288.2022.2107086

51. Introduction to the Americans with Disabilities Act. *ADA.gov*. October 4, 2024.
Accessed October 6, 2024. https://www.ada.gov/topics/intro-to-ada/

52. *PGA Tour, Inc. v. Martin*. (Supreme Court 2001). https://supreme.justia.com/cases/
federal/us/532/661/

53. *Urso v. Team Illinois Inc*. (Illinois Appellate Court 2024). https://ilcourtsaudio.blob.core.
windows.net/antilles-resources/resources/17df2403–28e6–43e0-af88-a5749f19a449/
128935_AEB.pdf

54. Beach MC, Price EG, Gary TL, et al. Cultural Competence: A Systematic Review of
Health Care Provider Educational Interventions. *Medical Care*. 2005;43(4). https://
journals.lww.com/lww-medicalcare/fulltext/2005/04000/cultural_competence__
a_systematic_review_of_health.7.aspx

55. Lal Shrivastava SRB, Shrivastava PS, Mendhe HG, Tiwade YR, Mishra VH. Cultural
Competency Training of Medical Students among Trauma Patients: Training and Assessment Strategies. *Journal of Pharmacy & Bioallied Sciences*. 2024;16:S1096-S1100.

56. Jongen C, McCalman J, Bainbridge R. Health Workforce Cultural Competency Interventions: A Systematic Scoping Review. *BMC Health Services Research*. 2018;18(1):1–15.

57. Association of American Medical Colleges. *Cultural Competence Education*. Published
online 2005. https://www.aamc.org/media/20856/download

58. Commission on Accreditation in Physical Therapy Education. *Standards and Required
Elements for Accreditation of Physical Therapist Education Programs*. 2023. https://
www.capteonline.org/globalassets/capte-docs/2024-capte-pt-standards-required-
elements.pdf

59. American Association of Colleges of Nursing. *Cultural Competency in Baccalaure-
ate Nursing Education*. 2008. https://www.aacnnursing.org/Portals/0/PDFs/Teaching-
Resources/Cultural-Competency-Bacc-Edu.pdf

10 Risk Management

Chapter Objectives: Following the completion of this chapter, the reader will:

1. Explain how risk management is optimally applied as a proactive strategy.
2. Recognize the steps and processes involved in developing policies and procedures.
3. Identify specific aspects of clinical practice that present liability risks.
4. Identify appropriate resources that are useful in developing risk management policies and procedures.

Risk Management

Risk management, as associated with sports or athletics, is often seen through the lens of managing the risk of specific injuries, and taking steps to reduce the risk of legal liability will also reduce the risk of injury to participants or patients. While specific injury risks do factor into the discussion, risk management involves much more than just trying to decrease the risk of a hamstring strain. Risk management includes developing and implementing best practices in all aspects of the health-care system in general, not just the risk of athletic injuries. Risk management also means identifying and taking all possible steps to decrease or eliminate any risk to athletes, patients, the clinician providing healthcare services, and well as the institution, clinic, or school employing the clinician.

Sun Tzu, a Chinese general and war strategist in, roughly, 500 BC, wrote "Attack is the secret of defense; defense is the planning of an attack"[1]. This is often paraphrased as the best defense is a good offense and it is appropriate when considering managing or controlling risk or liability. The very best defense against liability is to prevent the event in question from happening. To that end, good risk management strategies are spawned in good policy and procedure development. The untimely death of Drew Kleinknecht is an unfortunate illustration of this point.

Kleinknecht v. Gettysburg

On September 16, 1988, Lacrosse players on the Gettysburg College team were in off-season practice much like any other day. At some point during that practice,

DOI: 10.4324/9781003524823-10

defenseman Drew Kleinknecht stepped out of a drill and collapsed[2]. According to other players, Drew was not hit or involved in any type of collision prior to his collapse. Records of the rush of people working to get help for Drew are vague and it is difficult to determine exactly how long it was before it was determined that Drew was in cardiac arrest and the scenario was critical and life-threatening. Unfortunately, measures taken to save Drew at the hospital failed and he died later that day.

Two Gettysburg College coaches attended and supervised practice which was held on the softball fields just beyond the football stadium. Cour records indicate

> no trainers or student trainers were present. Neither coach had certification in CPR. Neither coach had a radio on the practice field. The nearest telephone was inside the training room at Musselman Stadium, roughly 200 – 250 yards away. The shortest route to this telephone required scaling an eight-foot high cyclone fence surrounding the stadium. According to Coach Janczyk, he and Coach Anderson had never discussed how they would handle an emergency during fall lacrosse practice.[2]

Gettysburg College should have had an emergency action plan in place to manage emergent care situations that arose during practices or games. At the time of Drew's death, Gettysburg College did not employ enough athletic trainers to ensure there was an athletic trainer at each practice for every sport. This fact only underscores the importance of having a plan in place which outlined, among other things, the roles and responsibilities of everyone, specific emergency equipment available, and specific details about how to initiate communication with emergency medical services.[3] Requiring all coaches and all on-field athletic department personnel would have ensured that those responsible for would have had the ability to perform basic first-aid and CPR. Perhaps the outcome would have been different, had steps been taken ahead of time to adequately train athletic department personnel.

In terms of positive outcomes, the event experienced by NFL Player Damar Hamlin on January 2, 2023, is on the opposite end of the spectrum compared to that of Drew Kleinknecht. Hamlin was struck in the chest at the exact instant when doing so could stop the heart, which it did. Unlike when Drew Kleinknecht fell incapacitated to the field, Damar Hamlin was assessed and immediately treated by certified athletic trainers.[3] Athletic trainers treating Damar had a well-developed and rehearsed plan for cardiac emergencies or other life-threatening events. Athletic trainers and other medical personnel executed the plan flawlessly with the player not only surviving the incident but returning to play the next year. There is little question that the emergency action plan previously devised, practiced, and implemented that day saved Hamlin's life.

Examination of these two scenarios provides a good starting point for discussing risk management. It is appropriate to begin the risk management discussion with policy and procedures. Facility design and management should also be considered when evaluating potential risks. In fact, every aspect of the system must be evaluated, including even, the actual healthcare delivery system itself including interaction with physicians and other providers.

Policy and Procedure

Policy and procedure differ in that policies are written expectations of behavior or actions and procedures are instructions for carrying out the behavior or action.[4] As previously mentioned in this chapter, risk management should include controlling risks for the clinician, the facility, the agency, or school, and the patient.

Guidelines published by the Board of Certification, Inc., include worksheets that can be used when writing policies and procedures. Areas in the risk management section of the guideline highlight the need to develop policy and procedures for safe practice in matters including, but not limited to:

- Inspection of facilities
- Emergency action planning
- Provision of care to visiting athletic teams
- Over-the-counter medication
- Drug testing
- Third-party billing

Resources for Writing Policy

The NATA Research and Education Foundation[5] and the National Athletic Trainers Association[6] partner to write and oversee the development of position statements on numerous topics of interest in clinical practice. These position statements serve as a valuable resource for professionals as policies and procedures are written. The topics covered by the positions statements include but are not limited to:

- Lightning Safety for Athletics and Recreation
- Environmental Cold Injuries
- Preparticipation Physical Examinations and Disqualifying Conditions
- Management of Sport-related Concussion (and 2024 updated Bridge Statement)
- Management of Asthma in Athletics
- Exertional Heat Illness
- Safe Weight Loss and Maintenance Practices in Sport and Exercise

Korey Stringer Institute

Korey Stringer was an offensive lineman who played for the Minnesota Vikings and died from an exertional heat illness in 2001. Since that time, the Minnesota Vikings, the National Football League, the National Athletic Trainers Association, and leading researchers in heat-related illness and injury partnered to establish and maintain the Korey Stringer Institute.[7] By conducting research and publishing educational material relative to heat illness and other potential risk areas, the Korey

Stringer Institute acts a valuable resource for policy development at all levels of athletics but has proven to be specifically important in providing education and advocacy in the secondary school setting. Policies recommended by the Korey Stringer Institute include the following:

- Sudden Cardiac Arrest
- Exertional Heat Stroke
- Traumatic Head/Brain Injury
- Exertional Collapse Associated with Sickle Cell Trait
- Lightning
- Asthma
- Anaphylaxis
- Spinal Cord Injury
- Preparticipation Physical Examinations
- Protective Equipment Fitting and Reconditioning

National Federation of State High School Associations

Comprised of individual state secondary school activities associations, the National Federation of State High School Activity Associations (NFHS) offers support for developing policies and procedures to protect student athletes through its Sports Medicine Advisory Committee (SMAC).[8] The NFHS prepares and disseminates position statements addressing numerous areas of concern specific to secondary school athletes. Some of the areas addressed include the following:

- Concussion Management
- Medical Devices
- Mouthguard Use
- Runner Safety
- Hydration
- Lightning
- Skin Infection
- Heat Illness Prevention

Facility Design and Operation

Areas of concern from a facility or agency perspective encompass everything from the visibility of patients within the facility to compliance with applicable electrical codes. While expertise relating to construction codes falls outside the scope of an athletic trainer, knowledge that any electrical outlets must be ground fault interrupter (GFI) compliant or having a policy for scheduled calibration and maintenance of therapeutic modalities does not. It is impossible to overplay the importance of sound risk management practices in facility design and operation. Regardless of whether it is working with existing facilities or engaging with architects and professionals as a facility is being designed and constructed, following best practices standards for minimizing risk can greatly reduce liability risks[5].

In documentation published by the Board of Certification, Inc., several specific areas for consideration in facility design and management are highlighted.[9] Facility design and/or operation should also be considered for protecting clinicians and patients from blood-borne pathogens as published by the Occupational Safety and Health Administration (OSHA). OSHA uses the term engineering control of blood-borne pathogen risks when discussing devices such as sharps containers and personal protective equipment such as gloves or protective goggles for the eyes.[10] Engineering control includes any piece of equipment or device that is used to control exposure to blood-borne pathogens and must be a consideration in facility design and operation as well as the purchase and availability of personal protective equipment.

Infrastructure for Risk Management

Traditionally, most athletic trainers were employees of colleges, universities, or secondary schools. Within that environment, the athletic trainer typically falls under the oversight of an athletic director. As the athletic environment in intercollegiate athletics and secondary schools evolves, this original system is coming under scrutiny. Coaches' salaries continue to rise, creating an environment in which, potentially, too much authority is given to an individual with an exorbitant salary but no medical expertise. It is, unfortunately, not uncommon for the interests of a multimillion-dollar-a-year coach to come into conflict with an athletic trainer working for a university.[11] The coach is paid millions of dollars to win games. The leap to "win at all costs" is not enormous when salaries are measured in millions. While many athletic trainers have reported coming under pressure from coaches, the situation within one of the premier athletic programs in the country actually resulted in an athletic trainer being released after coming into conflict with a coach. Karl Kapchinski, who is a certified athletic trainer, had worked for his alma mater for decades when he experienced conflict with a head coach who drew a multi-million-dollar salary. The conflicts eventually led to Kapchinski being dismissed.[12] In a phone conversation with Kapchinski (Karl Kapchinski, oral conversation, July 2024) he confirms there is always pressure to return players to the playing field. That's simply part of working with a patient population of elite intercollegiate athletes. Kapchinski, like most athletic trainers, reports at least some of the pressure is self-imposed. But the pressure should stop there. Athletic trainers must be free to make decisions completely outside of the influence of a coach. In what may herald a change of priorities, a team physician at a major university, dismissed after ongoing conflict with a coach, ultimately received a damaged award in excess of five million dollars.[13]

Rapp and Ingersoll[14] support transitioning away from the more traditional athlete healthcare delivery model which has existed for decades. In fact, such a move can be an effective step in reducing liability risks to both the clinician and the university. In a consensus statement published cooperatively by entities involved in athletic training, family medicine, orthopedic surgery, and interscholastic and intercollegiate athletics[15] it is strongly suggested that a patient-centered model of healthcare delivery is superior to traditional athletic department models and is, in fact, best practice. The following suggestions are made by the consensus statement:

- Athletic trainers work under the direction of a team physician based on their state practice act and professional standards.
- Athletic trainers follow policies and procedures that are written in conjunction with the team physician and supported by the school administration.
- Athletic trainers communicate return-to-play concerns with the team physician, with whom the final authority rests.
- All athletes undergo a comprehensive pre-participation physical examination and no athlete be allowed to practice or compete until documentation of the examination is provided.
- All schools with athletic programs have emergency action plans that are written, posted, and practiced by all who have responsibility for the acute management of athletes' injuries and illnesses.
- All schools have an appointed or designated team physician.
- All schools with athletic programs provide an adequate number of sports medicine providers, specifically and most appropriately athletic trainers, based on the number of athletic teams and athletes.

Risk management should be considered a proactive strategy, not a reactive strategy. While developing good policies and procedures such as emergency action plans will greatly enhance the quality of care delivered by a sports medicine team during the event, the real value of the plan or policy lies in prior preparation. Ensuring the plan is complete or that the policy meets current practice standards is a critical step in minimizing the extent of the damage when and if such an event takes place. As General Sun Tzu stated, planning an attack is the best defense!

References

1. Sun T. *The Art of War*. Filiquarian Publishers; 2006.
2. *Kleinknecht v. Gettysburg College*, 786 F. Supp. 449 (M.D. Pa. 1992). Justia Law. Published March 1, 2024. Accessed March 2, 2024. https://law.justia.com/cases/federal/district-courts/FSupp/786/449/1380085/
3. BillsTrainersCiteHamlinCaseasExampleforSchools,YouthLeaguestoMakeLife-Saving Plans. *AP News*. Published June 22, 2023. Accessed June 7, 2024. https://apnews.com/article/buffalo-bills-damar-hamlin-defibrillator-7b866eff65a02d2c61537284a7026436
4. BOCGuidingPrinciplesforATPolicyandProcedureDevelopment.pdf.
5. *NATA Research & Education Foundation—Supporting and Advancing the Athletic Training Profession through Research and Education*. Accessed June 2, 2024. https://www.natafoundation.org/
6. Practice & Patient Care. *NATA*. Published March 20, 2015. Accessed June 2, 2024. https://www.nata.org/practice-patient-care

7. Administrator. Korey Stringer Institute | Korey Stringer Institute. Published February 26, 2015. Accessed June 8, 2024. https://ksi.uconn.edu/about/korey-stringer-institute/
8. *Developing School Environmental Health and Safety Policies.* Accessed June 12, 2024. https://www.nfhs.org/articles/developing-school-environmental-health-and-safety-policies
9. BOCFacilityPrinciples.pdf.
10. 1910.1030 - Bloodborne Pathogens. *Occupational Safety and Health Administration.* Accessed June 8, 2024. https://www.osha.gov/laws-regs/regulations/standardnumber/1 910/1910.1030#1910.1030(b)
11. *Trainers Butt Heads with Coaches Over Concussion Treatment.* Accessed June 14, 2024. https://www.chronicle.com/article/coach-makes-the-call/
12. Halliburton S. Former A&M Athletic Trainer Says Coaches Forced Him to Clear "Good" Players. *Austin American-Statesman.* Accessed June 14, 2024. https://www.statesman.com/story/news/2016/10/12/former-am-athletic-trainer-says-coaches-forced-him-to-clear-good-players/9850329007/
13. Andrejev A, Williams J. Ex-PSU Doctor Awarded $5.25M in Suit Alleging Franklin Interference. *The New York Times.* Accessed June 12, 2024. https://www.nytimes.com/athletic/5529911/2024/05/30/penn-state-doctor-lawsuit-james-franklin/.
14. Rapp GC, Ingersoll CD. Sports Medicine Delivery Models: Legal Risks. *Journal of Athletic Training.* 2019;54(12):1237–1240. doi:10.4085/1062-6050-83-19
15. Goldenberg M, Adams KG, Anderson SA, et al. Inter-Association Consensus Statement on Best Practices for Sports Medicine Management for Secondary Schools and Colleges. *Journal of Athletic Training.* 2014;49(1):128–137. doi:10.4085/1062-6050-49.1.06

11   I Am Being Sued. Now What?

Chapter Objectives: Following the completion of this chapter, the reader will:

1. Define a claim and the associated steps one should take when being named as a defendant
2. Identify the process of retaining legal representation
3. Appreciate the role of an expert
4. Learn the basic components of a Deposition and a trial
5. Consider the possible outcomes following a lawsuit
6. Identify considerations for the continuation of professional practice

There isn't a person on earth who would enjoy being named as a defendant in a lawsuit. Simply put, it is not a fun experience no matter how you approach the situation. Let us begin this chapter in a unique fashion by sharing some key points for you to keep in mind right from the start:

- *Keep the news to an inner circle of trusted individuals*
- *Do not panic, instead remain calm with your thoughts*
- *Review your liability insurance policy*
- *Contact the appropriate stakeholders (lawyer, supervisor, etc.)*
- *Do not inappropriately access any documents related to the case*
- *Continue to do your job reliably and competently*

Being named in a lawsuit is rare, but common. What does this mean? It simply means that the number of athletic trainers named to defend themselves in a civil, or even criminal, case is composed of a very small percentage of individuals within the profession. However, there are enough that are named to merit everyone remaining cognizant of the process involved and of course methods to mitigate risk.

It is not possible to learn of being named in a lawsuit related to your role as an athletic trainer without having multiple immediate thoughts take over your mind. Do you even remember the situation? If so, how detailed can you recall all of the facts? Does it make you angry? Does it make you sick to your stomach? These are

DOI: 10.4324/9781003524823-11

just a few of the common questions you will ask yourself. Each person will react differently emotionally, some calm with a loss of appetite. Others may become angry and violent. One of the most important things you can do is rely heavily on your knowledge of what to do when you are named in a lawsuit. This chapter focuses on these very practical and necessary steps.

Defining a Claim

A claim is the official legal term used to describe the process sought to remedy a proposed wrong on the part of a party or parties and can be in the form of a civil or criminal matter. (Law.com, 2023) Athletic trainers are more likely to be named in a civil suit, whereas proven negligence seeks a verdict in terms of financial remuneration for resultant injury and damages. Additionally, if one is in fact found to be held negligent it is also possible that licenses, certifications, or memberships can be suspended or revoked. All findings and resultant outcomes are different from case to case.

How to Properly Respond to a Claim

As mentioned previously, learning about being named in a claim can create an unsettling feeling for any athletic trainer. This is an area very few athletic trainers have any experience with. Additionally, each case is different so any previous experience with a case may be of minimal value. Feeling uncomfortable, nervous, and even scared are all natural reactions to such a stressful piece of news. After all, you are being accused of contributing to the harm of another individual, and likely one that you were responsible for providing some form of care for.

The short answer to how one should respond to a claim includes collecting one's composure and creating a series of intentional steps that all contribute to one's response to the allegations (Superior Court of California, 2023). These steps will include the retainment of formal legal advice, limited conversations with trusted family and friends, and necessary conversations with your employer and their counsel. It is recommended to take careful notes from this point forward as it relates to any information and/or conversations that you have pertaining to the case.

The shock of being named in a claim can consume your thinking and challenge your ability to remain focused and move forward with your daily responsibilities to your job, family, and friends. Keep in mind that for one to be found negligent, an act of omission or commission must be proven with a preponderance of the evidence brought forth, including that you had an existence of duty to the patient, you breached such duty, the breach caused the injury, and physical and/or emotional harm resulted. Thus, you can initially play in your mind whether or not you think these can be shown. Regardless, one is always encouraged to remain calm and focused as a claim can take twists and turns ranging from being dismissed to going to trial.

Communicating With Appropriate Stakeholders

News of being named in a lawsuit is not the type of information you want to share on social media. It is best to keep conversation to a minimum and only include those that need to know. Keep in mind it is possible that if you are deposed and asked about the role you had in the claim, you may be asked about all of the people you talked to about the case since being informed and the nature of each conversation.

Family. Without question, most of us lean on family members during difficult times. It therefore would be normal human behavior for your first calls to be with your loved ones and those you trust most. In having conversations with these individuals, be sure to inform them not to share what you are telling them so that you can be assured information stays within a tight circle of individuals. This will prevent rumors from spreading, tampering with documents, and persuading of individuals involved in the case, and overall less drama for you as you journey through the process.

Lawyers. You will need legal assistance. Period. While some may have friends or family that are attorneys, it is wise to be sure that you are represented by counsel that has an understanding of what an athletic trainer is and does. In general it is better to have someone represent you that does not have a particular bias going into the case. Lastly, and likely most important, if you possess professional liability insurance you will be assigned an attorney as part of your paid coverage.

Employer. Communicating the information about being named in a lawsuit requires some careful thought about whether or not you share this information with your current employer. If the claim is based on an incident that took place with your current employer, in all likelihood they will have such knowledge. If so, then confirming your receipt of your legal notification is prudent. However, if the claim refers to a time when you worked for a different employer, you should seek the advice of your attorney as to whether or not you are required to inform your current employer. This will depend on the nature of the charges in the alleged claim as well as your contractual agreement with your current employer.

Insurance Company. Initially, the thought of contacting your professional liability insurance company may seem to be a negative action. You can be assured, however, that this call may be one of your most important calls and should happen as soon as possible. Any plan you have purchased will almost always provide you with an appointed attorney. This is one of the main reasons that you purchase professional liability insurance and it is important that you understand ahead of time what you paid for and what services are covered. It is through this relationship with your appointed attorney that you will receive legal guidance with all further communication and steps to defend yourself from the claim.[1]

Retaining a Lawyer for Representation

Because competent legal representation is of the utmost importance, assuring that one retains counsel is a critical first step to secure when being named in a claim. It is essential to understand the terms of your professional liability insurance and the terms of which a lawyer is appointed to you. In many cases, the professional liability insurance company will assign you a lawyer. The lawyer may be local to you, or come from a pool of people nationwide for them to choose from in their network. It is typically most beneficial if the lawyer assigned to you practices in the same state you live in or at least where the claim is being made for purposes of familiarity with jurisdiction law.

The inclination to simply sit back, listen, and adhere to any and all advice your appointed attorney provides you is very natural. But you must always remember you have a large stake in the outcome of the claim as it relates to your professional career and so you should be an active participant in the initial discussions with counsel. For example, it is essential that your lawyer understand what an athletic trainer is, the context of the claim related to your role as an athletic trainer, and especially if an expert can assist your defense to utilize your knowledge of identifying the most qualified expert to retain. Does your attorney know that certification as an athletic trainer entails and its scope or practice within your specific state licensure documents? Does your attorney understand what physician direction means? Is your attorney familiar with athletic training position statements? These are just a few questions that you would want answers to that will help you evaluate your attorney's knowledge of the claim as well as the need to retain a qualified expert. Typically, some education of what you do as an athletic trainer will need to be done in the context of the claim so the attorney can appreciate the details. It is reasonable for you to be expected to do some educating relative to the role and scope of practice of an athletic trainer, however, you should not have someone representing you that truly is completely unaware of athletic training as a profession.

What You Need to Know About Professional Liability Insurance

People possess different views as to whether or not athletic trainers should possess their own professional liability insurance. Some may feel as though the coverage they have from their employer protects them adequately. To those who believe such is the case, be sure you actually know what the employer's coverage entails and exactly how you will be covered. Are there any scenarios where your alleged wrongdoing will influence an employer's legal team to suggest what you may have done was outside of the scope of your terms of employment and therefore they will opt not to represent you? It is vital to understand that lawyers employed by a company are paid to represent and defend that company, not you specifically. Your defense is not their first priority! Others have even gone as far as to suggest it is better not to have your own professional liability insurance because if you do you can be sued for more money, even though it is paid through the insurance company. The belief here is that you are "worth suing." If you are covered by your employer, always check to see if that will also provide protection for you when working per diems for activities that are not part of your primary employment setting.

When you consider the annual cost of a policy, the services provided by most professional liability insurance plans are well worth the investment of the safety net they provide. Simply put, if you are sued, and have no insurance coverage, you will find yourself paying for all expenses out of your pocket. Attorney fees can rise to hefty amounts very quickly. Ask yourself honestly if you were named in a lawsuit, are you prepared to finance your own defense? It doesn't matter if you are innocent of the alleged claim or not. You will still need to be represented by someone in the legal system to navigate you through the process. This is no time to play lawyer and believe that you have the expertise to defend yourself like you may have done defending a speeding ticket in traffic court.

Where does one begin when considering a policy? Sometimes the simplest method is to ask colleagues about their experiences with their policies. Do not be surprised if most are unable to tell you details other than it was easy to purchase and they never really had to use it. That is not the advice you should settle on. Speak with the different providers, find an athletic trainer who has in fact had to put their policy in play, and ask for their candid experiences. Some policies may be recognized through a sponsorship of one's professional association, but keep in mind such sponsorships are not necessarily based on quality of coverage or services. Instead, they are purchased relationships to help brand the policy provider. Some general yet important items to consider in purchasing a policy include the following:

- Cost of the policy
- Type of incidents covered under the policy
- Amount of coverage for each type of incident
- Length of coverage time
- Dates of active coverage
- How are attorneys identified
- How are experts identified
- Does the policy provide coverage outside of the United States
- How does a policy apply to duel credentials
- Does the policy require an additional rider and fees to cover substance abuse, acts of sexual offenses

Perhaps one of the most confusing areas to evaluate is the two general types of defined coverages: claims made and occurrence. In simplest terms, each is described as follows:

- Per Claims Made—Your coverage is only activated when you file a claim during the policy period. If your policy is canceled for any reason, you will not be insured at the time of a claim.
- Per Occurrence—Your coverage applies if the incident occurred while your policy was active. This is most beneficial when claims are filed at a later date, but you were insured at the time of the alleged wrongdoing.

Discovery Process

Discovery is a legal process where both parties, plaintiff and defendant, request documents and relevant information from each other or from third parties. The purpose of discovery is to gather as many of the facts as possible to better understand the full nature and complexity of a case. This process may be quite lengthy and take months to even years, in some cases. Examples of information that may be gathered include but are not limited to medical notes, images, and results of any tests performed such as X-rays or MRIs, verification of licenses, background checks on individuals, emails, phone records, seeking of qualified expert witnesses, questioning of associated parties through the legal process of depositions, and anything else that attorneys deem relevant to fact find. Any documents requested during discovery are often done so through a subpoena and are required to be provided by law.

The Deposition Process

Most who have had the experience of being part of a legal deposition will tell you it was not fun and likely one of the most terrifying and nerve-wracking experiences of their life. Being on the receiving end of a deposition is not something athletic trainers do every day. One can be asked to take part in a deposition as a defendant or a possible witness to the facts. Typically, attorneys will gather as much information as possible prior to asking a defendant to be deposed. Once asked under subpoena to be deposed, one has no choice in whether or not to participate. Depositions are considered to be a part of the discovery process, where in addition to gathering facts by questioning witnesses and the defendant, attorneys can cross-check statements with existing facts that have already been gathered. A deposition usually takes a few hours but in some cases can last a few days in a complex and detailed case.

It goes without saying that an athletic trainer will not likely have experience with depositions. In all cases, the assigned, or as is more commonly referred to, "retained," lawyer will prepare you as best as possible for the deposition experience. As a named defendant, you will be subpoenaed by the plaintiff's attorney. While the experience may be stressful, it is your opportunity to tell the facts under oath according to how you recall them. Your attorney will guide you as to overall demeanor and responses to questions for example should you not recall the exact fact pattern or sequence of events. Some general basic advice[2] that can be utilized during depositions are as follows:

Always prepare and follow your attorney's guidance

- Do not memorize any testimony, rather be familiar with the facts
- Always be truthful. If you do not know or recall a fact, state it as such and do not guess
- Refer to documents whenever possible to state absolutes
- Maintain a professional demeanor at all times, avoid combative responses
- Avoid responding to hypothetically posed questions
- Be consistent in your responses
- Dress professionally

Keep in mind that traditional depositions would take place in person with lawyers from both sides present. Additionally, a stenographer who records all of the questioning and testimony will be present. Prior to the start, an oath will be taken whereby you will swear to tell the entire truth at all times during the deposition. You may be given breaks, for example, every hour, at which time you will be reminded upon return that you remain under oath. The deposition can take in any of the lawyers' offices, or in some cases can actually occur at your place of employment. Additionally, a video recording may be requested in which case there will be additional individuals present to provide professional-level video testimony of the entire deposition. In recent years and especially during the COVID-19 era, many depositions were taken virtually through a secured connection. This format certainly cuts down on expenses associated with any travel for any of the parties. However, it requires a slightly different method for preparation so one is comfortable in this type of approach.

A Settlement in a Case

A settlement is an outcome whereby both sides of the case come to an agreement that essentially puts an end to the claim. With a settlement comes concessions from both sides. Such concessions may include but are certainly not limited to any of the following:

- A public statement used by all parties
- An agreement to keep any and all information sealed with no further disclosure of any information
- Reporting of wrongdoing of one's state regulatory board and/or affiliation with memberships that require certain ethical behaviors[3]
- A financial award

A settlement will very likely create mixed emotions. For most, the end of the process provides some relief and allows for one to move forward with life. The outcome of a settlement may leave one slightly confused and even with an empty feeling. In other words, the ending of the claim may occur without one being found negligent or with the full ability to clear one's name. Quite often, lawyers with the majority of input from one's liability insurance company will agree to a financial settlement amount that is, in their view, fair and less costly for them as compared to going to a trial. This is not a negotiation process you, as a defendant, will have a voice in. An example of this is if an athletic trainer were named as a defendant in a personal injury claim. Let's assume the plaintiff was seeking damages of $250,000 for a sustained injury that prevented him from playing college sports and with physical and emotional challenges. After months of discovery, neither side's legal representation believes this number is fair and reasonable; however, neither side wants to take a chance and go to trial and completely lose their case. The sides might go back and forth with their discussion and point of view as they see the case until an agreement is reached. The insurance company may agree with the lawyers and settle on an amount of $90,000. This may anger you because if you feel you did no wrong and you don't want to see the plaintiff be rewarded. Keep in mind much of this will also go toward paying the attorneys. You must always keep in mind that the legal system is far from perfect, and more times than not a settlement will be reached to avoid a costly and timely jury trial.

Participating in a Trial

When a claim is not settled a trial date will be set where the plaintiff will be tasked to prove their claims in front of a judge and jury. Trials can be brought to civil or criminal court, with the overwhelming majority of athletic training claims being of the civil nature. As previously described, the outcomes of a civil trial may result in sanctions and fees, and require a preponderance of the evidence to be proven for an athletic trainer to be found negligent. On the contrary, a criminal case may result in probation, incarceration, and hefty fees. For one to be found to be criminally neglected the facts must be proven beyond a reasonable doubt.

During the trial, the athletic trainer will take the stand under oath in a court of law and be directly examined by their own attorney as well as cross-examined by the plaintiff's attorney. It is also during the cross-examination where the plaintiff's attorney will attempt to identify inconsistencies in responses as well as compare statements made in one's previously completed deposition. Taking the stand in a courthouse will likely be a very intimidating experience. Once again, it is important to maintain one's composure and always state the truth and the facts as they are known.

Career Continuation

Being sued may be one of the most challenging times in one's otherwise rewarding career as an athletic trainer. The thoughts, speculation, anxiety and so much more will likely play themselves out in one's mind in so many different ways and times. This may make it difficult to focus and move on with life, at both work and home. It is not uncommon for one to begin to question one's own knowledge and skills and have doubts at times about their ability to perform tasks competently.

Perhaps the single, most important thing one can do is make every effort to focus on returning to one's normal life as soon as possible. The discovery process can take some time, and the unknowns of the developments of the findings in a case can truly wreak havoc on one's mindset. Nonetheless, allowing additional stress to overwhelm you can lead to alterations in your behaviors, how you treat others, and potentially your work performance. You can be more guarded, less trusting, and more conservative in your interactions and patient interventions. Essentially, doubting yourself and being fearful of wrongdoing or failure. While you may have learned some things throughout the process, it is imperative to not dwell on the claim itself. There will be vital times when you will need to focus on the case and reflect on the facts as part of your defense preparation. Aside from those times, assure you are working with confidence and integrity and restore outlets in your life to maintain a satisfying life–work integration that best fits your style.

References

1. Law.com | The Premier Source for Global Legal News & Analysis. *Law.com*. Accessed October 16, 2024. https://www.law.com
2. Konin JG, Ramey M. *Becoming an Expert Witness in Health Care and Litigation: A Beginner's Guide*. Routledge; 2024. doi:10.4324/9781003522744
3. nata-code-of-ethics.pdf. Accessed October 16, 2024. https://www.nata.org/sites/default/files/nata-code-of-ethics.pdf

Index

Note: Page numbers in *italics* indicate figures.

ableism 83–84
Amateur Sports Act (1978) 74
American Medical Association 8
Americans with Disabilities Act (ADA) 83
Annual Football Fatality Survey 69
Anti-Defamation League 82
antisemitic speech 82
APA Dictionary of Psychology 80, 83
athletic training: credentialing and
    regulatory processes 7; governing
    agencies 7; regulatory requirements
    in 7–8
autonomy 19–21, 41

Beauchamp, T.L. 19
beneficence 21
Board of Certification (BOC) 7, 10, 51;
    Code of Professional Responsibility 46,
    79; Practice Analysis 6; Standards of
    Professional Practice 2, 46
breach of duty 9
burns 70–73

case law 3–4
cause-and-effect relationship 10
Center of Excellence on LGBTQ+
    Behavioral Health Equity 82
Childress, J.F. 19
Civil Rights Act: Title IX (1964) 23; Title
    VII (1964) 82, 83
civil trial 103
claims 97; career continuation 103; civil
    trial 103; legal representation 98–99;
    respond to 97
clinical practice: application in 11–12;
    documentation types 49–51;
    gender-based discrimination 80

Cohen v. Brown University 81
collegiate athletic setting 61–63
commission/malfeasance 9
Commission on Accreditation of Athletic
    Training Education (CAATE) standards
    6, 49, 76, 79, 84
concussion 55–56, 63, 68–69
confidentiality 22; case study 23;
    compliance 10
confirmation: verbal *vs.* written 30
consensus statements 45, 46, 94
Corbo v. Garcia case 72
coverage 11; types of 100
COVID-19 pandemic 36, 82, 102
cultural competency training 84

*Davis v. Monroe County Board of
    Education* 81
deception 34
deposition process 101–102
disability 83–84; categories 83
discovery process 100–101, 103
discrimination 3–4, 23–24, 79–80; case
    study 24, 85; disability and ableism
    83–84; ethnicity 81–83; gender- and
    sex-based 80–81; LGBTQ+ Community
    82–83; mitigation strategies 84–85;
    racial 81–83
documentation 10–11, 48–49; case study
    52; clinical notes 49–50; continuing
    education requirements 51; daily
    sign-in logs 50; emergency action
    plans (EAP) 51; injury reports 50;
    insurance information 50; inventory
    reports 51; issues within 17; medical
    referral forms 50; patient-rated
    outcome measures (PROMs) 50;

policy & procedure manuals 51;
    treatment/rehabilitation plans 50;
    types of 49–51
drug testing 73–74
duty to care 9
duty to inform 36

emergency action plans (EAPs) 1, 11, 51,
    90, 94
emergent situation informed consent
    37–41
employer-sponsored coverage 11
Equal Employment Opportunity
    Commission (EEOC) 82
ethics: in healthcare 19; medical (*see*
    medical ethics)
ethnic discrimination 81–83; *see also*
    discrimination
Eveland *vs.* City of San Marcos case 57
evidence-based medicine: and standard of
    care 45–47
exertional heat illness 69–70

falls 74–75
Family Educational Rights and Privacy Act
    (FERPA) 10, 51
Feleccia v. Lackawanna College
    11–12, 58
Fenster, D. 72
Fourth Amendment of the Constitution 73

*Gebser v. Lago Vista Independent School
    District* 81
gender-based discrimination 80–81; *see
    also* discrimination
Good Samaritan Law 11
governing agency 7
gross negligence 1, 58, 59; *see also*
    negligence

Hamlin, D. 90
harm to plaintiff 9; cause-in-fact of 10;
    proof of proximate cause of 9–10
hate crimes 82–83
healing art 55
healthcare ethics 19; *see also* ethics
healthcare providers 7, 8, 65; ethical
    codes of conduct 23; racial
    discrimination 82; recruitment
    and retention efforts 84; sound
    documentation practices 48
Healthcare Providers Service Organization
    (HPSO) 71

health inequities 79
Health Insurance Portability and
    Accountability Act (HIPAA) 10, 51
Human Rights Campaign 83

inclusive healthcare system 82, 84
Indiana State High School Activities
    Association 70
informed consent 8, 28–29; components
    of 29–30; document for research 37,
    38–41; emergent situations 37–41;
    practical examples 35–36; during
    pregnancy 34; types of 31–33; verbal
    34; written 31, *31–33*
Ingersoll, C.D. 25, 93
Institute for Healthcare Improvement
    (IHI) 79
insurance: company 98; documentation
    50; liability 11; professional liability
    99–100
intercollegiate athletics 25, 58–63, 93
International Olympic Committee
    (IOC) 74

Kapchinski, K. 93
Kleinknecht v. Gettysburg College 4,
    89–91
Knapp, N. 21
Korey Stringer Institute 91–92
Krueger, C. 20
Kruger v.San Francisco 49ers 20, 36

Lackawanna Junior College (LJC) 58
lawsuits 4, 65, 97; employer notification in
    98; falls 74–75; infections incidence 64;
    secondary school setting 55; treatment
    for injury 62
lawyers 63, 98–99
legal liability 2, 89; *see also* liability
Legal Shield 6
legal terminology 3
Legal Zoom 6
LGBTQ+ Community: discrimination
    82–83
liability 8; defense against 89; insurance
    11, 98–100; reduction strategies 10–11;
    study of 2
licensees: sound judgment 24
Lindsay, S. 83
locality rule: standard of care 44
*Lopez v. Metropolitan Government of
    Nashville* 81
Lu, D.W. 80

malfeasance 9
malpractice 8–10, 71
Max's Law 56
medical documentation 3
medical ethics 19; autonomy 19–21;
    beneficence 21–22; confidentiality
    22–23; discrimination 23–24;
    non-maleficence 21–22; role fidelity
    24–25; scope of practice 24–25
medical malpractice 9, 43, 62
medical referral forms 50
medicolegal issues 3–4
Minnesota Vikings 69, 91–92
misfeasance 9
mitigation strategies: discrimination
    84–85

National Association of Intercollegiate
    Athletics (NAIA) 63
National Athletic Trainers' Association
    (NATA) 8, 11, 45–47, 51, 79, 91;
    Best Practices Guidelines for
    Athletic Training Documentation 48;
    Code of Ethics 2, 23; LGBTQIA+
    Advisory Committee 82, 84; position
    statements 9, 45–47, 51, 91;
    Research and Education Foundation
    (Foundation) 45, 46, 91; Support
    Statements 45
National Collegiate Athletic Association
    (NCAA) 23, 69, 73–74
National Federation of State High
    School Activity Associations (NFHS)
    92–93
National Football League (NFL) 20, 21, 64,
    69, 70
negligence 9; breach of duty 9; cases
    11–12; clinical case study 15–16; coach
    actions 1; duty to care 9; failing to hire
    qualified medical personnel 11–12;
    failure to assess and evaluate concussion
    symptoms 12; failure to report head
    injury symptoms 12; fundamental
    components 9–10; harm to plaintiff
    9–10; malfeasance 9; misfeasance 9;
    nonfeasance 9
nonfeasance 9
non-maleficence 21, 22

Occupational Safety and Health
    Administration (OSHA) 93
Olympic Charter 74
omission/nonfeasance 9

paternalism 19–20
patient-rated outcome measures
    (PROMs) 50
PGA Tour Inc. v. Martin 84
Pinson v. State 12
position statements 9, 45–47, 51, 91
professional liability insurance
    98–100
professional sports setting 64
*HR734 Protection of Women and Girls in
    Sports Act of 2023* 83
proximate cause of harm 9–10
*Putman v. Board of Education of Somerset
    Independent School* 81

racial discrimination 81–83; *see also*
    discrimination
Rapp, G.C. 25, 93
recklessness 1, 58, 59
regulatory requirements: in athletic
    training 7–8
rehabilitation clinical setting 64–66
return-to-play (RTP) decision 19,
    35–37, 57
Riley's Rule 11
risk management 4, 10–11, 66, 89;
    facility design and operation 92–93;
    infrastructure for 93–94; policy and
    procedure 91–92
role fidelity 24–25

Schwartz, M.R. 82
scope of practice 8, 24–25; Rule No.
    64B33–4.001 76
secondary school setting 54–58, 92
second impact syndrome 44
setting-specific risk: intercollegiate setting
    58–63; professional sports setting 64;
    rehabilitation clinical setting 64–66;
    secondary school setting 54–58
settlement 102–103
sex-based discrimination 80–81; *see also*
    discrimination
sexual harassment 3–4, 80
Sim, J. 19
Smith, A.D. 82
Snyder, C.R. 82
SOAP (subjective, objective, assessment,
    plan) notes 49–50
sound documentation practices 11, 48, 51;
    see also documentation
Sports Medicine Advisory Committee
    (SMAC) 92

Sports Medicine Licensure Clarity Act 7
standard of care 3, 8, 20, 54, 55;
    challenges 43; evidence-based
    medicine and 45–47; locality
    rule 44; position and consensus
    statements 45
Strategic Alliance 7–8
Stringer, K. 69–70, 91–92
supervision 75–77
systemic inequality 82

Terry, H.T. 43
tort 8–10; categories 8–9; intentional 8;
    negligent 9; strict liability 9

Trentley, C. 80
trials: civil and criminal 103

undue influence 36–37
United States Olympic Committee (USOC) 74
Urso v. Team Illinois, Inc 84

verbal informed consent 34; *see also*
    informed consent

Williams v. Athletico 12, 55
Winkelmann, Z.K. 10
written informed consent 31, *31–33*;
    see also informed consent

For Product Safety Concerns and Information please contact our EU
representative GPSR@taylorandfrancis.com
Taylor & Francis Verlag GmbH, Kaufingerstraße 24, 80331 München, Germany

www.ingramcontent.com/pod-product-compliance
Lightning Source LLC
Chambersburg PA
CBHW060321220326
41598CB00027B/4387

* 9 7 8 1 6 3 8 2 2 0 6 3 3 *